Home Care for the Elderly

HOME CARE
—— FOR THE ——
ELDERLY

An International Perspective

ABRAHAM MONK
—*and*—
CAROLE COX

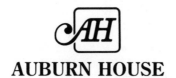

AUBURN HOUSE

New York • Westport, Connecticut • London ©1991

Library of Congress Cataloging-in-Publication Data

Monk, Abraham.
   Home care for the elderly : an international perspective / Abraham
Monk and Carole Cox.
   p. cm.
   Includes bibliographical references (p.) and index.
   ISBN 0–86569–005–7 (alk. paper)
   1. Aged—Home care—Cross-cultural studies. I. Cox, Carole B.
II. Title.
HV1451.M66 1991
362.1′4—dc20   90–1280

British Library Cataloguing in Publication Data is available.

Library of Congress Catalog Card Number: 90–1280
ISBN: 0–86569–005–7

First published in 1991

Auburn House, 88 Post Road West, Westport, CT 06881
An imprint of Greenwood Publishing Group, Inc.

Printed in the United States of America

The paper used in this book complies with the
Permanent Paper Standard issued by the National
Information Standards Organization (Z39.48–1984).

10 9 8 7 6 5 4 3 2 1

Contents

Preface

The demand for home care services for the frail aged and the disabled has been growing relentlessly in recent years. Several factors have contributed to this trend. First, the practice of institutionalization in nursing homes, which intensified during the last quarter century, is now giving way to a more balanced consideration of alternative home-based services. Second, the prohibitive cost levels of nursing homes as well as the increase in the number of the elderly, particularly those in the eighty-five and older age bracket, have also stimulated interest in home care services. In addition, new technological advances have led to the production of smaller, portable equipment that can be brought into the patients' homes, obviating the need for longer hospital or nursing home stays.

Home care is regarded as either a substitute or an alternative to nursing homes. The latter view—namely, that it constitutes an option within the continuum of long-term care services—tends to be gaining greater credence. In both cases, the underlying philosophical premise has been that ill and disabled persons have the right to be cared for, whenever possible, in their homes.

The shifting interest towards home care for the elderly may be traced to the 1965 Medicare Amendments (Title XVIII) of the Social Security Act and the resulting multiplication of home health agencies. The number of such agencies grew from 252 in 1966, to an estimated 10,000 in 1986, with 50 percent of that increase taking place after 1982.

Regrettably, this rapid process occurred without comprehensive planning or a careful anticipation of forthcoming trends. Services were set up in a reactive fashion, and home care evolved as a patchwork of fragmented and disjointed programs. This is explained, to a large extent, by the fact that services are based on several streams of funding, with disparate restrictions and variations in eligibility.

The search for a more viable and coherent model of home care prompted the Administration on Aging of the United States Department of Health and Human Services to examine successful program experiences and innovations in other parts of the world. This book is based on the results of a study of home care services in six countries—Argentina, Canada (Manitoba), England, the Netherlands, Norway, and Sweden—funded by the United States Department of Health and Human Services, Office of Human Development Services, Administration on Aging (OHD AoA 90–AR–0109—01), with additional support from the Abrons Foundation. It was conducted between September 1987 and June 1989 by the two authors with the cooperation of a team of local researchers in each of the countries.

The countries in reference were selected after a preliminary review of policies, organizational structures, and creative solutions to problems of service delivery in many nations. As a single-perspective study, it selectively screened out community and home care from a broader array of elderly-related services. Yet it aimed to treat the subject matter in a systemic way by constantly relating it to its broader policy and cultural underpinnings.

This book summarizes the main results of this inquiry. The findings are not intended, however, to be used as instant prescriptions for replication. Their significance rests more on the holistic portrait of how six countries wrestle with the demand for home care than on the presentation of piecemeal methods and techniques.

The introduction (Chapter 1) begins by briefly reviewing the extent of the need for home care in the United States, the scope and types of services, their operational modalities, and their policy frameworks. Chapter 2 describes how the data were collected and analyzed. Chapter 3 places home care in each country's policy context. Chapter 4 reviews how home care services are organized and operated, and Chapter 5 focuses on the recruitment, training, and utilization of personnel. Chapters 6 and 7 screen outstanding innovative programs and practices, and Chapter 8 analyzes evaluative and advocacy trends. The book concludes in Chapter 9 with a summary of the findings and suggests the possible adaptation to the United States of innovative practices identified in the study.

Acknowledgments

Numerous persons and institutions offered advice and assistance that enabled us to complete this project.

We wish to express our appreciation to the study's advisory committee members Camilla Flemming, Robert Hoyer, Bill J. Halamandaris, Linda Hoffman, Janet S. Sainer, and Bernard Warach.

To the international research correspondents, we owe much gratitude. They include Catherine Thompson in England, Kees C. Knipscheer in the Netherlands, Betty Havens in Canada, Svein O. Daatland in Norway, Gerdt Sundstrom in Sweden, and Mario Strejilevich and Mirta Zatelli in Argentina.

We also appreciate the assistance of others involved in gerontology and elderly care, such as Harold Sheppard of the International Exchange Center on Gerontology at the University of South Florida in Tampa; Charlotte Nusberg of the International Federation on Aging and Marla Bush of the Administration on Aging, U.S. Department of Health and Human Services (USDHHS), both in Washington, D.C.; Kirsten Milbrath of the Amherst Senior Center in Amherst, New York; Rosa P. Resnik of Seton Hall University in South Orange, New Jersey; and Theresa Martico-Greenfield of the Jewish Home and Hospital in New York City.

For their help at Columbia University's Institute on Aging, we would like to thank research assistants Judith Whang and Jacqueline Berman as well as administrative aide Linda Nye.

We are grateful, too, for the funds to execute the project, which came from two sources, the Administration on Aging in the Office of Human Development Services at USDHHS, and the Abrons Foundation.

Finally, our special appreciation is reserved for the dozens of individual interviewees and public and voluntary organizations in the six countries on which the book focuses. These persons and groups shared with us their knowledge, experience, and insights, making the entire project possible.

1

Introduction: Home Care in the United States

NEED FOR HOME CARE

It is estimated that about 5 million chronically ill elderly living in the community are in need of at least minimal assistance to perform their activities of daily living (U.S. Government Accounting Office [GAO], 1986). By the year 2000, over 15 million older persons will suffer at least one chronic illness that will limit their functioning, a 50 percent increase over the estimates for the 1980s (Spiegel, 1987). While studies continue to demonstrate that most assistance is currently provided on an informal basis by family and friends, the growing number of single or childless older adults, the simultaneous aging of family members along with their frail relatives, and the shrinking of the pool of women care givers will exacerbate the demand for more formal home care services. This is confirmed by the fact that in fiscal year 1985 Medicare paid about $1.7 billion for home health care services, more than six times the amount spent in 1976 (GAO, 1986).

Another key factor impacting the home care industry has been the 1987 changes in hospital discharge policies. A year-long study by the Senate Special Committee on Aging revealed that Medicare's newly adopted prospective payment system of DRGs (Diagnosis Related Groups), which requires hospitals to discharge patients at an earlier stage of convalescence, places an additional stress on posthospital services (Special Committee on Aging, 1986). Almost simultaneously, New York State's Medicaid case-mix reimbursement system, Resource Utilization Groups (RUGS), has limited the access to nursing homes for those patients not requiring intensive skilled nursing care. Similar case-mix reimbursement systems adopted by other states (Maryland and Ohio, among others) have also led to an increased demand for home care.

In New Jersey, a state which has had the prospective payment system in effect since 1980, the total admissions and home health agencies increased by 48 percent between 1980 and 1983 (Taylor, 1986). National data on the utilization of home health services similarly reveals a substantial growth in use following the implementation of the Medicare's Prospective Payment System (PPS) policies. Visits per user, total number of visits, and visits per 1,000 Medicare enrollees rose from 17 per 1,000 in 1974 to 46 per 1,000 enrollees in 1983 (Leader, 1986).

It is not surprising that the home care industry has been expanding to meet the demand for services. During the twenty-year period between 1967 and 1987, the number of Medicare-certified home health agencies rose from 1,753 to 5,877 (National Association for Home Care, 1987). With this phenomenal rate of growth, expenditures by Medicare on home health care doubled between 1980 and 1983, from $772 million to $1.5 billion, growing at an annual rate of approximately 34 percent per year (Doty, Liu, and Weiner, 1985). By 1985 it had already become a $9 billion industry, and it positioned itself as the fastest growing segment of the $400 billion health care market (Nassif, 1986–87). Moreover, it is expected to double in financial volume to $18 billion by the year 1991. This expansion has not occurred uniformly across the country. New York State alone absorbs 70 percent of the Medicaid funds earmarked nationally for personal home care services.

Despite this overall budgetary increase, services do not seem to keep up with the presumed need. Denials by Medicare for home health services reimbursement have also multiplied. Medicare-covered visits rose an average of 19 percent between 1980 and 1983 but slowed to only an 8 percent increase in 1984 despite the fact that the demand for services under the prospective payment system continued growing (Heinz, 1986). As a result, many consumers must pay for the services themselves or do without care.

TYPES OF SERVICES AND AGENCIES

There is considerable variation in the types of services provided by home care agencies as well as among the agencies themselves. Services may range from sophisticated technological care, usually offered by a hospital, to assistance with household tasks such as cleaning and shopping. The scope of services provided includes personal care with medical supervision and assistance, personal maintenance, rehabilitation, and social and emotional counseling. Ancillary community services, such as meals-on-wheels and transportation programs, may also be considered a part of home care.

Home care is provided by four types of agencies: public, nonprofit, proprietary, and a mixed type of dual sponsorship. All public agencies operated by state or local governments usually fall under the jurisdiction of health and welfare departments. Nonprofit agencies include organizations such as the Visiting Nurse Association and its multiple affiliates, religious denominations, hospitals, nursing facilities, and rehabilitation programs. Proprietary agencies are operated for profit, while combined agencies may be sponsored jointly by a governmental and a voluntary unit such as in the contractual association of a health department and a Visiting Nurse Association.

The wide array of services that an individual may require and the assortment of providers that may be involved in the provision of care can be complex and confusing. It is not always clear which services are essential for the independent functioning of the individual and who should be responsible for providing and coordinating the services.

Home care agencies may also be classified according to whether or not they are Medicare-certified. As the number of certified agencies has expanded, there has been an even more accelerated growth of the uncertified ones, so that the two types are now approximately equal in number. This process may partially result from the fact that denials by Medicare for home health services have continued to escalate, causing many persons to pay privately for care. Moreover, many persons exhaust their Medicare benefits and continue on a custodial private-pay basis. In addition, many of the noncertified agencies receive state funding under Title XIX, Title XX, and Title III programs, which also provide homemaker and home health aide services.

Certified and uncertified agencies differ along the types of services they operate. They do not uphold the same standards for supervision, personnel requirements, or record-keeping and training methods. Whereas those which are Medicare-certified must adhere to specific guidelines in these areas, the same is not true for those which are uncertified. As of 1988, less than 2 percent of the uncertified agencies have been accredited by the National Homecaring Council, a division of the Foundation for Hospice and Homecare. This accreditation is contingent on adherence to basic standards and guidelines for services.

Many states have developed their own administrative guidelines for home care agencies that receive state funding. For example, the Iowa legislature has established rules that place the burden on the provider agency to assure that homemakers and home health aides receive adequate training. Alaska and New Jersey require agencies receiving state funds to either meet accreditation standards or specific state requirements. New York, Connecticut, and Florida have instituted licensure laws for non-Medicare agencies and paraprofessional staff.

ACCESS TO HOME CARE

Referrals for home care services may come from many sources. Most commonly, they are made by hospital discharge planners, physicians, social service agencies, families, or the patients themselves. However, if services are to be reimbursed under Medicare, the person's need for service must be documented by a physician.

ASSESSMENT IN HOME CARE

Once a request for services is made, home care personnel proceed to assess the intended user's needs and capabilities. Initially, this evaluation is meant to establish both eligibility for coverage within policy guidelines and the package of services required. Reassessments are usually made at regular intervals to ascertain whether changes have occurred in the person's condition and whether the services meet the needs and standards of care.

Since hospitals are a primary source of referrals to home care, the physicians, nurses, discharge planners and social workers are often the ones who make the initial assessments. The inherent problem in these hospital-based assessments is that they seldom take into account the home environment or the availability of pre-existing community supports.

CAAST is an example of a patient assessment method commonly used by attending physicians to determine the need for home care (Glass and Weiner, 1976). It covers the following five areas:

1. *Continence.* Fully continent / incontinent for two days to one month / incontinent for more than one month

2. *Ambulation.* Fully ambulatory / unable to move independently more than 20 feet two days to one month / unable to move for more than one month

3. *Age.* Younger than 65 / 65–79 / older than 79

4. *Social background.* Admitted from home and likely to return home / admitted from an extended care facility and likely to return there / admitted from home and likely to be discharged

to an extended care facility / admitted from extended care facility and likely to be discharged to another

5. *Thought processes.* Fully oriented / disoriented for more than one month

Each of these items is scored from 0 to 2 based on severity and weighted for chronicity. A higher total score indicates greater dependence in posthospital care and the need for more extensive posthospital arrangements. The assessment is based closely on a medical orientation and does not collect data on social functioning, emotional needs, or wishes of the patient. These are often the precipitating factors leading to the institutionalization of the elderly.

Bulau's (1986) assessment form for use by home health agencies expands the traditional medical orientation by including data on the patient's social needs and functioning. It records whether the applicant

1. is homebound;

2. is under care of a physician;

3. needs part-time or intermittent skilled nursing services and at least one other therapeutic service, for example, physical or occupational therapy;

4. experiences medical, nursing, and social needs that can be met adequately by the home health care agency in the applicant's place of residence.

It also determines whether the home health care services are necessary and reasonable for the treatment of the applicant's illness or injury.

The workers' qualifications constitute a perennial concern in the maintenance of the quality of home care. Regrettably, a substantial volume of care is provided by unlicensed paraprofessionals performing the roles of homemakers and home health aides. These workers are employed by social services and welfare and health departments as well as by proprietary agencies. They generally receive perfunctory training, if any. Their compensation rarely exceeds minimum wages levels—and may even, due to few fringe benefits, slide below. These workers have little opportunity for advancement. In addition, they rarely receive continuous and direct supervision. These inherent problems affect the overall quality of the care.

The Omnibus Budget Reconciliation Act of 1987 has attempted to rectify some of the problems associated with quality of care. It included provisions to protect the rights of recipients of services of home health agencies, to strengthen certification procedures, and to specify training requirements for personnel.

CARE PLAN

Once the staff (a supervisor, nurse, etc.) has determined that the needs can be adequately met through their home care program, they proceed to outline a care plan. This plan spells out the range of services, the amount and duration of each service, and the balance between informal and formal care providers. The objective here is to define what is the minimum amount of service required to maintain the person at home.

Care plans also constitute the framework for monitoring both the client and the quality of care. They are, therefore, essential for evaluating a program's effectiveness. The Home Care Quality Assurance Act of 1987 requires that agencies develop care plans that identify required services, provide a means for identifying additional client needs, and include coordinating mechanisms with other service agencies.

SERVICE DELIVERY

Three dominant categories of personnel are involved in providing home care services. Home health care registered nurses generally make the initial and subsequent evaluations of nursing needs. They also provide specialized nursing services and report to the home care agency and physician of changes in the client's status. The nurse, in most instances, is the supervisor of the other home care staff.

Home health aides assist with personal care and toileting, bathing, simple medical procedures, ambulation, and exercises. They may also oversee the administration of medications.

Homemakers are responsible for housekeeping, meal preparation, laundry, grocery shopping, and help with household-related duties. Their work may also entail companionship, but it does not encompass personal care that must be provided under nursing supervision.

Other skilled services commonly offered through home care include speech therapy, physical therapy, and occupational therapy. These are often contracted with other agencies, with the home care supervisor monitoring the participation of the required specialists.

COORDINATION OF SERVICES

Considering the wide array of services in the home care field, the need for coordination is evident. It may be hampered, however, by variations in agency philosophies regarding service provision, differences in assessment procedures, separate and often conflicting plans for care, differing perspectives on the kind and amount of services required, and disagreements about the type of personnel best suited to provide those services (Trager, 1980).

Another inherent problem is deciding who should act as the service coordinator among the staff of these diverse programs. A lack of such service articulation can result in duplication of services and manpower, poor service accessibility, and the underutilization of services.

Increasingly, case managers are stepping in to assist with the coordination of services. The responsibility of the case manager is first to ensure that proper services are provided and then to keep track of the various providers. This can involve explaining the total plan to the patient and the family, monitoring daily activities, evaluating services, solving problems, and acting as a liaison between the client and agencies. However, the effectiveness of the case manager's role is limited when the providing agencies remain independent and are under no mandate to accept the manager's plans.

THE EFFECTIVENESS OF HOME CARE

Measuring the effectiveness of home care services is as intricate an issue as the very nature and organization of the programs themselves. Criteria as to what constitutes effectiveness vary according to the philosophies and interests of the participating agencies. However, under current government funding and guidelines, the cost savings or efficiency criteria become the overriding concerns when comparing home care to other forms of care.

A recent study (Bergner et al., 1988) of home care for patients with chronic lung disease found that after one year there was no difference in survival, pulmonary functioning, or everyday functioning for those receiving care from respiratory home care nurses, standard home care, or those getting care in the physician's office. However, the cost of the respiratory home care was significantly higher than the other modes of treatment, such as those offered in physician offices or hospitals.

A study comparing home dialysis provided by home health aides with traditional hospital-based dialysis also casts doubt about the cost effectiveness of providing specialized technical care at home (Sparer et al., 1983). The findings reveal no differences in hospitalization or mortality rates between those receiving home care dialysis and those receiving traditional hospital dialysis. However, the training of the dialysis aides brought the cost of the home care to a level comparable to the cost of hospital dialysis in half of the experimental clients. These findings tend to indicate that if cost-effectiveness and savings are the main objectives of home care, it may be necessary to target services on persons requiring less costly care. Home care does not appear, therefore, to be the universal panacea.

Another approach to evaluating home care is to focus on its impact on institutionalization rates. An evaluation of a comprehensive coordinated home care program in Chicago found that an experimental group receiving home care experienced a significant reduction in nursing home admissions compared to controls who did not receive the service (Hughes, Cordray, and Spiker, 1984). The experimental group also had an increase in their sense of wellbeing and a decrease in their unmet needs for community services. However, the mortality and hospitalization rates for the two groups did not differ.

An extensive comparison between nursing home and home care patients based upon samples from twenty home health agencies and forty-six nursing homes in twelve states was made by Kramer, Shaughnessy, and Pettigrew (1985). Their findings indicated that home care patients were younger, had shorter lengths of care, and were more functionally independent than nursing home patients. Among the Medicare patients in each program, the home care patients showed greater improvement in independent living skills. The author concluded that home care may be most cost-effective as a substitute for acute care following a hospital stay.

Capitman (1986) reviewed the extensive evaluations of five demonstration projects in long-term care sponsored by the Health Care Financing Administration (HCFA). The five projects were the New York City Home Care Project, the Long-Term Care Project of North San Diego County, Project OPEN, the South Carolina Community Long-Term Care Project, and the On Lok Community Care Organization for Dependent Adults. All of the demonstrations offered (1) expanded case management; (2) paraprofessional home health services to meet needs associated with activities of daily living, instrumental activities of daily living, and mental status disabilities; (3) multidimensional assessment and reassessment and service arrangement and management.

The programs differed in both their target populations and objectives. The South Carolina program attempted to divert nursing home applicants to home care, while On Lok provided a consolidated package of care to individuals who would otherwise be admitted to nursing homes. The other three projects succeeded in upgrading, through additional services, the home care packages provided to Medicare recipients.

The results of the evaluations suggested that expanded home care services and case management may only impact on nursing home use when they are offered to persons who have made nursing home applications, having no noticeable effect on equally frail persons who have not made such applications.

Other outcome measures that have been used in evaluating the effectiveness of home care programs include patient satisfaction and degree of dependence on the service. Bass and Rowland (1983) studied two home care programs in the Boston area that provided general homemaking and domestic services. The data, collected from 750 clients with an average age of seventy-eight years, showed a high satisfaction with the service, although the degree of dependence on it was less certain. Only one-third felt that they would be unable to live independently without it.

Client satisfaction with a professional home health care team has also been examined (Zimmer, Groeth-Juncker, and McCusker, 1985). The team consisted of a physician, geriatric nurse practitioner, and social worker, and it targeted only clients who were seriously or terminally ill. The findings indicated that the target group had fewer hospitalizations, nursing home admissions, and outpatient visits than the controls not visited by the team. Although the clients did not differ from the controls on morale, both they and their care givers were more satisfied with their care than those not receiving home services.

Conclusions regarding the effectiveness of home care services are difficult to make on the basis of these studies alone. However, even with diverse clienteles, home care appears to be associated with higher client satisfaction and a reduction in the use of nursing homes. The issue of cost-effectiveness, particularly for those requiring highly specialized technological care, needs to be more closely examined, and perhaps balanced with other evaluative criteria. The effect of home care on care-giver stress and burden, as well as its relationship to the care givers' ability to continue maintaining the person in the community similarly require further scrutiny.

PUBLIC POLICY ON HOME CARE

The diversity found in the myriad services and providers in the home care field reflects, to a large extent, the lack of unified or consistent public policies. Although the federal government aims to reduce health care costs by means of earlier discharges from hospitals—the DRGs—this has not resulted in increased funding for home care services. The absence of a comprehensive policy in this area has led to confusion among both agencies and consumers, as both are unclear regarding reimbursable or entitled services.

The Medicare Catastrophic Coverage Act that went into effect in January 1989 did extend home care benefits under Medicare but not to the degree needed to fully legitimize community care as an alternative to institutionalization. Moreover, the act's continued focus on medical diagnosis as the main prerequisite for benefits ignored many of the social and emotional problems associated with the maintenance of the chronically ill person in his or her home. With the repeal of the act several months later, those limited gains were also curtailed. Four federal programs provide most of the current public funding for home care: Medicare, Medicaid, Title XX, and the Older Americans Act.

MEDICARE

Although home health care constituted only about 4 percent of the total Medicare expenditures in 1987, this program remains the largest source of public funding for home care. Moreover, the home health care benefit is the fastest growing benefit in the program. Sections 1814 and 1861 of the Social Security Act require Medicare Part A reimbursement for the medically reasonable and necessary care of homebound Medicare-eligible beneficiaries who are in need of part-time or intermittent skilled nursing, physical therapy, speech therapy, occupational therapy, medical social services under the direction of a physician, medical supplies and equipment, and part-time or intermittent services by a home health aide, as authorized by regulations and the medical services of interns and residents under an approved teaching program of a hospital.

The lack of clarity of some of the program's regulations was bound to create confusion. The absence of standardized definitions for "medically reasonable and necessary," the basic requirement for establishing care, led to a certain degree of arbitrariness in the decisions to reimburse or decline many claims. The Omnibus Budget Reconciliation Act of 1987 brought about more explicit definitions of "homebound" and "intermittent care." "Homebound" is thus defined as not being bedridden but needing assistance or support to leave home due to an illness. "Intermittent care" is care provided for a maximum of thirty-eight days, seven days a week. Services may be extended under "exceptional circumstances," a concept that remains undefined.

Bills for payment of home care services are processed for Medicare by ten fiscal intermediaries throughout the country. These third-party payers consult with the home care agencies, do billings, collect payments, and conduct audits and evaluations. They are also under a mandate to "administer the program in a manner that achieves maximum savings and cost avoidance for the Medicare trust funds" (Federal Register, 1986). This latter requirement often places them in a relentless adversarial and restrictive rather than balanced relationship with the provider agencies.

Cost controls, as reflected in the denials of claims, are in fact a major source of concern to the home health agencies. Since the initiation of Medicare's prospective payment system the number of denials rose from 1.2 percent in 1983 to 8.3 percent in 1987 (National Association for Home Care, 1988). At the same time the HCFA, which administers the program, attempted to eliminate the "waiver of liability" under which the home health agencies were given flexibility in interpreting Medicare rules and regulations. The waivers allowed persons whose eligibility was questionable to receive services. Under the waivers, an agency with fewer than 2.5 percent of its visits disallowed in a quarter is permitted to be reimbursed for services found not to be covered at a later time. HCFA, however, did not succeed in its attempt and these waivers were extended to 1990.

The increasing attention being paid to long-term care insurance and extended health coverage may begin to reshape the government's attitude and policy towards home care benefits under Medicare. Changes likely to occur are the coverage of other than medical or skilled nursing care, such as homemaker services, dietary and prevention counseling, respite care, and case management. The inclusion of these services would expand the role and effectiveness of home care in meeting many of the pressing and chronic needs of the elderly.

MEDICAID

Medicaid (Title XIX of the Social Security Act) is a joint federal and state program that provides medical assistance for low-income persons. Each state administers its own program subject to federal guidelines, which mandate that it be provided to recipients of Aid to Families with Dependent Children and those receiving Supplemental Security Income, a program intended for the blind, disabled, and aged. However, states have the latitude to determine the scope of benefits and level of reimbursement.

Medicaid must cover home health care physician services. It must also provide intermittent or part-time nursing care, home health aide services, and medical supplies and equipment. As in the Medicare program, these services can be provided only after the written recommendation of a physician, and the plans must be reviewed every sixty days.

Under the system of Medicaid waivers, the states are able to provide community and home services to persons who would otherwise be placed in an institution. The waivers broaden the range of services that can be provided, including social and personal services and case management. States are also permitted to offer homemaker, home health aide, and chore services; rehabilitation; day health care; and respite care. However, the costs of these home care services must not exceed the cost of Medicaid care in an institution.

Waivers are a small part of the Medicaid program, and when requesting them, states have to provide assurance of decreased state expenditures for home care services. This requirement, combined with the cost-containment objectives, have inhibited a wider use of waivers. It is difficult to prove in all cases that the home care costs less than a nursing home, or that a recipient would end up in an institution if home care services were not available.

SOCIAL SERVICES BLOCK GRANT—TITLE XX

Title XX, the Social Services amendment to the Social Security Act, is the major social service program funded by the federal government. Under this grant states are permitted to allocate funds for services that may prevent or reduce inappropriate institutional care. Title XX thus authorizes home health, homemaker, chore, and home management assistance. It also provides for adult day care, home-delivered meals, transportation, counseling and prevention, and social support services. States, however, can use the Title XX funds on any services they select. Funds are allocated on the basis of population within a federal budget ceiling. Because competition for funds within the states' programs is great, its impact on home care services has been limited.

OLDER AMERICANS ACT

Under Title III of the Older Americans Act, grants are given to state Agencies on Aging, which are responsible for funding the local area Agencies on Aging in their planning, coordinating, and advocacy of services for older persons. Congress has given priority under Title III to in-home services such as homemaker and home health aide care, friendly visiting, and telephone reassurance. Case management, case assessment, adult day care, and respite care may also be provided. Many states coordinate these programs with those of Title XX.

FUTURE DIRECTIONS

As the demand for comprehensive long-term care services increases, home care services are expected to similarly expand. A primary concern is to develop a coherent federal policy that provides a framework for this growth.

Data carefully documenting needs and costs—including unmet needs—as well as the effects of home care on delaying institutionalization among comparable groups of elderly and its effects on care givers, must be collected to shape that policy. While it is true that expensive hospital-type services may not be cost-effective when provided at home, it's important to realize that this type of care is not needed by the majority of persons targeted to receive home care services. Most could benefit from simple domestic assistance, which would foster their independence and help to maintain them in the community. Once home care is viewed as a means not only to attain a humanitarian goal but also to bring health care costs down to manageable limits, its role in long-term care policy and services may be more firmly legitimized.

Policymakers interested in creating more effective home care programs may benefit from learning about current international experiences. The six countries selected for this study are known for the salient role that home care services already play in their communities. A critical examination of their accomplishments may therefore serve as a model for improving services in the United States.

2

The Conduct of the Study

This study focused on the experience of six countries known for the prominent role they assign to community-based services as well as for their record of innovativeness in home care. The countries—England, Norway, Sweden, Argentina, Canada (province of Manitoba), and the Netherlands—were selected as a result of literature searches and consultations with international organizations and coordinating bodies in the fields of gerontology, health, and social services; national professional organizations; and gerontological researchers in several countries.

The initial number of targeted countries was larger than six but was narrowed down due to time and budgetary constraints. Those selected met the following three criteria: (1) evidence of substantial commitment to community service strategies, (2) a fairly high degree of experimentation with new service models, and (3) the adoption of public policies specially focused on home care service solutions. There was also the underlying expectation that the selected countries had approached home care in different ways and that they would exhibit a distinct range of model solutions. This expectation could not be fully realized, but the results were not disappointing, either. Even countries with similar public policy traditions and backgrounds, known to have historically initiated and borrowed from each other, proved to be quite different and to have followed opposite courses of action when confronting analogous social problems. Moreover, countries that began with the same policy objectives and service philosophies ended up forging different programs, more attuned to local conditions and idiosyncracies. There are, in essence, uniquely culture-bound components in all service models, as well as more generic elements that may lend themselves to transferability beyond their national boundaries.

The overall goal of this study was to precisely apprehend and understand the gist of those foreign solutions. It then sought to identify the program features that could eventually be considered for adaptation in the United States.

More specifically, this study had the following aims:

1. To collect and synthesize information on the planning, operation, and delivery of innovative home care services

2. To assess the potential transferability of successful foreign initiatives

3. To design a conceptual model or models of home care services that may help integrate those foreign experiences into existing programs in the United States

4. To translate the research findings into practice guidelines that will assist home care agencies in the testing and adoption of these innovations

This latter research dissemination objective required the enlistment of several national umbrella organizations, direct providers in the voluntary sector, and governmental agencies involved in the provision of home care.

METHODOLOGY

There were seven major stages in the implementation of this study. The first was the formation of an advisory committee made up of leaders in the home care field. These persons assisted in identifying problems and strategic issues in the provision of services. The advisory committee included representatives of the following organizations:

1. National Association for Home Care

2. Foundation for Hospice and Home Care

3. New York Foundation for Senior Citizens, Inc.

4. Jewish Association for Services for the Aged

5. New York City Department for the Aged

6. New York City's Human Resources Administration.

In addition to highlighting topics in home care that merited international inquiry, the representatives of these organizations also assisted with:

1. designing the questionnaire,
2. reviewing the drafts of findings, and
3. making suggestions for adaptations to programs in the United States.

The second stage involved the cooperation of both the International Federation on Aging and the International Association of Gerontology. These agencies advised in the selection of researchers in each of the six countries. The chosen specialists were all closely involved with the field of long-term care and specifically with home care services. They were designated as research correspondents and played critical roles in the following tasks:

1. Reviewing the initial interview guides
2. Making recommendations regarding content areas
3. Translating the instrument into Spanish (in Argentina) and summary guidelines of the questionnaire into Norwegian and Swedish
4. Producing lists of potential interviewees
5. Making all necessary contacts for the actual interviews
6. Sending out the questionnaires in advance and in preparation for the meetings
7. Organizing the research schedules and itineraries
8. Escorting the senior researchers to many of the interview sessions and facilitating with translations when needed

The research correspondents also collected background documents on their respective home care programs, policies, previous research reports, and so forth, and enabled the research staff in New York to prepare preliminary literature reviews. Finally, they reviewed and critiqued the reports of findings. The names and affiliations of research correspondents are acknowledged in the preface.

The third stage of the project was concerned with the finalization of the instrument for the interviews. Based upon previous research as well as the input of the advisory board members and the research correspondents, the instrument focused on the following areas:

1. *Definition of home care services*:
   What services constitute home care?

Are there regional or local differences in home care services?
Are there different levels of home care such as intensive nursing care and light housekeeping tasks?

2. *Determination of need for services*:

Who makes the assessment for care?
How are appropriate services decided upon?
Is there a specific assessment instrument that determines the older person's need for care?
Are there eligibility requirements to qualify for home care?

3. *Administration of home care services*:

How are health and social service needs integrated and funded?
Are all services administered through one agency?
How are services between agencies coordinated?
What are the alternatives to home care services?

4. *National policy*:

Is there a national policy governing home care services?
How much flexibility is there in this policy?
What proportion of persons are not receiving home care services but should be? Is there adequate coverage?
Is there equity between regions in the country?

5. *Home care and hospital care*:

How does home care integrate with hospital care?
Who arranges for home care services after discharge from the hospital?

6. *Reasons for home care services*:

Is home care seen as preferable to institutional care?
Is home care preferred because of an inadequate supply of other services or beds in institutions?

7. *Family and home care*:

What is the role of the family in home care? How involved do they have to be?
Does the family have to make a financial contribution?

8. *Funding home care*:

Are services paid for out of tax revenues?
Do individuals have to contribute?
Are all types of services covered? If not, which are covered and which are not?
Is there a limit to the length of time that services may be obtained without payment?
How does the cost of home care compare to institutional care?

What is the average cost per month for a home care recipient?
Are tax incentives or payments given to families caring for elderly at home?
How are services paid for—by the visit, hour, day?

9. *Quality of care*:

Who monitors the quality of the services?
What rights do recipients have regarding their assessments of care or complaints with services?
Is there one set of standards that serve as the basis for assessing quality?
Are standards determined on a national basis, or are there regional or local standards for care?
What types of records are maintained on each patient?
How much personal care is given as compared to respite care for the care giver?

10. *Licensure*:

Are all home care agencies licensed by the government?
Are there national regulations regarding home care services?
What types of records or reports are required by the agency?

11. *Manpower*:

Who authorizes home care services?
What is the role of physicians in home care? Do they review records?
What is the educational requirement for home care workers?
What types of personnel are involved in providing services?
What are the tasks of each type of care worker?
What strategies and inducements are used to recruit and retain home care workers?
What is a description of the typical worker?
How are workers paid? Hourly, daily, benefits?
Who supervises the workers?
How many patients does a worker have to see?
Are there enough workers to meet the home care needs?
Who is actually the employer?
Who trains the workers?
How extensive is the training?
What difficulties, if any, are there in retaining personnel?
Is there a career advancement ladder for personnel?
Are there any home care jobs that persons refuse to take?

12. *Evaluation*:

What process is used to evaluate the home care services?
How are individual workers evaluated?

What indicators (mortality, morbidity, functional improvement, life satisfaction, cost savings, etc.) are used in evaluating the service?
Are comparisons made between programs?
How are innovations in one program or in one region shared with other home care agencies?

13. *Problem and issues in home care:*

What are the main problems associated with the delivery of home care service?
Is patient abuse ever a problem? If so, how is it dealt with?
Are there problems of physical or financial exploitation?
How are the agencies addressing these problems?
What changes are anticipated in services?

These topics reflected the main concerns of professionals involved in home care programs in the United States. It was not anticipated that each of the persons interviewed would be knowledgeable about every topic, but this comprehensive framework provided assurance that significant data would not be overlooked.

The foreign researchers identified the items most pertinent for the interviews with each prospective respondent. The interviews were conducted during the months of June, July, and August of 1988, with Dr. Abraham Monk doing the interviews in Sweden, Norway, and Argentina and Dr. Carole Cox doing those in the Netherlands, Great Britain, and Canada.

The fourth stage took place prior to the field trips for data collection. It consisted of the review of the literature collected by the foreign correspondents and through the bibliographic searches conducted by the New York research staff. These documents served as a basis for the field interviews and were incorporated into the final report.

The fifth stage consisted of the actual field interviews in the six countries. A total of 140 face-to-face sessions, often involving more than one person, was held. These interviewees occupied many levels and positions related to home care, ranging from state ministers to service consumers. Information was gathered from government officials, elected policymakers, agency administrators, direct service providers, advocacy groups, researchers, and consumers.

As stated, the interviews were not necessarily held on an individual basis. On many occasions, an appointment with a single respondent resulted in a collective session with the entire departmental or division staff of a public or voluntary organization. Some of these meetings involved up to twenty-three participants in open and extensive discussions on a specific issue raised by the interviewer.

The sixth stage involved the integration of the data collected in the interviews with agency and government documents, new literature, and the initial literature review. Interview data was transcribed by questionnaire items, compared for commonalities, and summarized. In several instances, translations of corroborating documents were commissioned to check the validity and reliability of interview material or simply to update the information collected.

The seventh and final part of this effort was the review of foreign models and the preparation of a working summary of innovations in home care that highlights their most successful objectives and experiences. Based upon this data, guidelines and recommendations for services were developed for programs in the United States.

The initial concern that a standardized research instrument may not be applicable to all countries was not substantiated. It proved to work well, although slight differences of emphasis or focus, depending upon each country's policy and services context, had to be introduced. As an example, most countries visited had not yet formulated quality-of-care standards and licensing requirements. They were not particularly concerned with estimating unit-of-service costs or evaluating intervention outcomes, and thus questions in these areas did not yield much data. There was more to learn, instead, from the resourcefulness and flexibility of their home care programs.

The researchers were mindful that the solutions generated by each country are consistent with their particular value systems, type of government, economic conditions, and long-standing ground rules for public decision making. Each country had its unique blend of normative principles and administrative traditions. Furthermore, each may define a set of priorities that is of little relevance to other countries. Suggestions to transfer innovations must consequently remain sensitive to special national circumstances and avoid the temptation of literal adoption.

This study selectively screens out community care and home care for the elderly from the broader spectrum of gerontological services. It treats the subject matter in a systemic way, however, by constantly referring it to its broader policy and cultural underpinnings. It also aims to follow a "double mirror" perspective, that is, once a major innovation is identified, it should be contrasted with conditions prevalent for analogous situations in the United States. If something works elsewhere, the first question is, Would it work here too, once the local circumstances are taken into account?

Even when an innovative practice is recommended, its adoption is bound to entail distortions or to require adjustments. The innovation is re-created when it blends with the new host culture. Furthermore, the analyst-researcher may deliberately modify the innovation to ensure a better fit. The second question then is, Granted that it works elsewhere, how should the idea be reshaped to ensure that all or some aspects of it may work here too?

CONCEPTUAL MODELS

Three conceptual models were used to design this research. The first, derived from Smith's model of the policy implementation process, consists of five elements (1973). It begins by identifying the idealized policy, that is, the optimal end result that policymakers aim to achieve. It then defines the target group, the population that stands to benefit or to be affected by the policy. Consideration is given here to assessment, eligibility, and qualifying requirements for obtaining benefits or services. Next, the implementing organization is identified. This study took into account the range of concurrent implementers—public agencies at all levels of government, contract agencies, private sector providers, and so forth. It considered their specific domains or responsibilities as well as their interactions and coordinative processes.

The fourth component relates to the environmental factors, that is, all the societal, political, and economic elements that have a stake in or may be influenced by the policy. Finally, once the idealized policy is being carried out, new tensions and conflicts may surface in this environment. They reveal inadequacies that need to be discussed, transacted, and negotiated. This becomes the final stage of feedback and policy reformulation.

The second conceptual framework that influenced this study's design was derived from the Forecasting Model for HCFA Long-Term Care Programs, produced by ICF, Incorporated (1979). It consists of six elements or modules:

1. *Impairment module.* Identification of the population at risk and in need of services.
2. *Eligibility module.* Income and entitlements of the population at risk.
3. *Demand module.* It includes the range of services offered by the program under scrutiny as well as the patterns and trends in requests for services.
4. *Supply module.* Regulations restricting or facilitating service provision, reimbursement rates, and types of service.
5. *Utilization module.* Actual usage, length of use, and linkage or transfer to other services.
6. *Expense module.* Costs, reimbursements, budgeting, and financing considerations that ensure the program's continuity.

Although basically an economic model, the HCFA model provided some elements that were incorporated in this study's guidelines.

The third and final model was developed by the researchers to compensate for some of the gaps contained in the two preceding models as well as to introduce a greater degree of specificity. The model includes the main themes or categories spelled out in the preceding research instrument, as follows:

1. Definition and rationale for services
2. National policy
3. Assessment of need
4. Administration
5. Coverage
6. Funding
7. Manpower
8. Quality of care
9. Evaluation
10. Licensing
11. Coordination with hospitals and other services

Models, or abstract representations of reality, are often used for explanation and for integrating new knowledge. The findings of this study, as presented in the following chapters, are largely explained and organized along most of the dimensions or categories of the third model described above.

3

The Public Policy Framework

National policies in the six countries tend to express a preference for community home care over institutional care. This is usually justified on moral, philosophical, and economic grounds. There is, however, a concurrent realization that home care cannot always replace institutional care.

All national policies seem, therefore, to acknowledge that there are complex cases of multiple chronicity that can no longer be attended in the home environments. This realization occurs—in some countries—when the cost of home care surpasses comparable care in a nursing home. Yet even this threshold may be disregarded if the care is terminal or required for a short period of intensive convalescence. There may, in fact, be no defined point at which institutional care is actually preferred over home care. The pragmatics of each case or situation as well as established precedents determine the course to follow.

This chapter reviews governmental policies toward home care in each of the six countries. It also examines the context in which those policies are promulgated and the roles performed by different levels of government in the planning, operation, monitoring, and funding of home care.

NORWAY

Norway is a sparsely populated country. It has a population density of twelve people per square kilometer as compared to 230 per square kilometer in Great Britain. One third of Norway is located north of the Arctic Circle, but this area is home to only one-twelfth of the population, less than 400,000 people. The country's population is concentrated, for the most part, in large urban centers, but a substantial minority remains scattered over great distances, clustered in small hamlets, rural villages, and coastal towns.

Norway has experienced in recent decades a marked increase in the proportion of old people. The total population has grown from 3.3 million in 1950 to 4.1 million in 1980. However, the cohort of persons sixty-seven years of age and older nearly doubled in that same period, from 268,000 to 525,000 people.

By 1980, one out of every eight Norwegians had reached the pensionable age of sixty-seven, but the ratio is expected to narrow to every seventh person by 1990. Further projections indicate that this proportion will level off and remain stable until the early part of the twenty-first century. By 2025, every sixth Norwegian will be sixty-seven or over. Similar to the United States, the Norwegian old-old cohort, composed of those who are eighty-five years of age and older, is experiencing the largest demographic expansion, while this age group also has the highest incidence of chronic and disabling conditions causing dependency. The high rate of urbanization and residential mobility have scattered family members of different generations, leaving many elderly alone and isolated in the rural countryside. With the increase in the number of women entering the labor force, many of these traditional care givers are no longer necessarily available to care for the old.

Public Policy

Norway is an advanced welfare state that earmarks a substantial portion of its public budget for health and social services. Taxation is also high, as is public consumption compared with most other Western societies, but private consumption is fairly low. Of the 33 billion kroner spent in 1982 on the elderly—about 9 percent of the gross national product—19 billion, or almost 60 percent, were income transfers, mostly pensions. The 14 billion balance was spent on health and social services.

These services are for the most part publicly financed. Some health and social institutions are privately owned by nonprofit organizations, but even these are also largely subsidized by public funds. Most of the latter abide by the same regulations and standards set for the publicly owned institutions.

Norway has adopted a decentralized system of government that relies primarily on the local or municipal level for the provision of major services. There are, in fact, 453 such "communes" or municipalities. These are clustered in a second level of nineteen county or departmental units called *Fylke*. The third and highest level of public administration is the central or state government. It sets general policies and awards block grants to the other two levels of government, but it does not prescribe what programs they should institute, nor does it determine how they should prioritize among competing service claims. The central government also administers the national health insurance and income maintenance programs for the aged and disperses funds for health service delivery to the other two levels of government.

Each of these three levels of government—the municipality, the county, and the central government—must meet the budgetary requirements for all services under its jurisdiction. The population pays taxes to all three of them. The central government collects the bulk of income taxes, but part of these revenues are shifted back to the counties and the municipalities. Moreover, the counties are also assisted by the national health insurance fund to operate hospitals and related medical services. To compensate for potential inequities in the provision of services that may result from disparate tax levies—some municipalities and counties are wealthier than others—the central government allocates a series of block grants according to a population formula. This equalization policy takes into account the proportion and number of children and elderly people in each political jurisdiction, as well as its tax base. Obviously, the intent of these block grants is to offer a minimum floor of services. As a result, some counties and municipalities are generously assisted while others receive almost nothing, given the tax revenues they already collect.

Social Service Legislation

The 1969 Act of Parliament that regulates hospital and specialist health care delegated to the counties the administration of both general and mental hospitals, the planning and provision of medical specialist services, and the provision of services to older persons and long-term care patients in hospitals.

The municipalities' responsibilities in the health domain are defined in the 1982 Commune Health Services Act. Local governments are required to provide general medical services, including medical rehabilitation and physiotherapy; nursing care, including health visitor and home nursing services; old age homes; and home help services. Many have added service centers, similar to the American concept of multiservice senior centers.

As of January 1988, municipalities began paying wages and providing respite care for family care givers of dependent relatives. In addition, they included nursing home care under their jurisdiction. In 1991 they will also be responsible for the services for developmentally disabled persons.

The growing concern over health care led to the presentation by the executive branch of government to the Parliament, in 1987, of a white paper outlining strategies to improve health services. This paper recommended comprehensive policies for health promotion and prevention, including a five-year plan aimed at reducing rates of cancer, heart and circulatory diseases, accidents, and suicides. It also outlined the rehabilitation of the handicapped and comprehensive care for the aged.

The latter recommendation is predicated on the prevailing philosophy that services for the aged client should be offered in the person's habitual environment and that relocation to restrictive institutions should be avoided. The number of nursing home beds for the population eighty years of age and older, which as of January 1988 stood at 22.7 per hundred, is expected to be gradually reduced. The central government's intent is to have part of the resources currently allocated to nursing home care eventually shifted to community-based services.

The very mission and identity of nursing homes are expected to change. These institutions will eventually evolve into a flexible service pool adapted for the provision of home care, sheltered housing and group living services, and of course long-term institutional care. In its minimalist definition a pool consists of a home nurse, a general practitioner, and a social worker. The home nurse ensures continuity of care and a de facto case management function. The other two team members act as backup consultants or specialists.

This model of services varies, of course, from municipality to municipality. An additional principle being advanced is that home services should foster the active involvement and financial compensation of family care givers. It is argued that such a solution is economically sensible because it ends up costing less than nursing home care, and it also gives families an incentive for undertaking a prolonged and demanding role. It is recognized, however, that institutional care will always be needed and that family care is not a universal panacea.

The Decentralization Model

Norway's decentralization model of government leaves for the most part the pragmatics of service delivery to municipal authorities. They are required by state law, however, to provide health and social services. While there is no specific legal mandate for home help, virtually all have such services. The central government also recommends standards of desirable quality of service, but municipalities are not bound to adopt them. The Norwegian Association of Local Authorities accepts technical assistance from the central government, but reserves for its affiliates the right to make their own choices. In theory, Norway may therefore be characterized as a federation of 453 autonomous governments, some consisting of no more than a few hundred residents and each designing its own system of services. In practice, however, there is a fairly high degree of conformity with governmental recommendations and borrowing from each other's experience. The result is a de facto standardization. The important feature is that standardization is not imposed from above.

Decentralization also implies that municipalities will distribute services along smaller geographical subdivisions easily accessible to service recipients. The concept, however, goes beyond the creation of reduced catchment areas. In the particular case of the aged it also aims to (1) do away with the distinction between institutional and home care; (2) facilitate a more flexible linkage between agencies, professionals, and auxiliary personnel; and (3) deliver services by teams of workers rather than by solo practitioners.

Another concurrent objective of the decentralization strategy is that all services be offered, whenever feasible, in one place and by multidisciplinary teams. This should facilitate easy access to the consumers' providers. Ideally there will be a single provider, similar to a case manager, for each client, or at the maximum two to three providers. It is hypothesized that this greater individualization will reduce waiting lists and long waiting periods. Above all, it is expected that the new system will tear down absurd compartmentalizations between services and inconsistent eligibility rules.

Home Care Services

Home care consists of two specific services: home help and home nursing. The first, home help, is by far the largest service offered to the aged in Norway, based on the number of persons reached. Its aim is to offer assistance to the elderly and disabled who otherwise would be unable to continue living at home. The home help service includes light housework, shopping, laundering, meal preparation, window washing, and related daily tasks. Although home help is not restricted to the elderly, they are the primary users of the service.

Home nursing is the fastest growing form of home help, and it serves as a viable alternative to institutionalization for those elderly who need low-level medical treatment and/or supervision. As with home help, home nursing is not age-specific, but most patients are over the age of sixty-five. The types of services available through the home nursing program are information and counseling, curative treatment, rehabilitation, and general nursing.

SWEDEN

Sweden has one of the world's highest ratios of old people relative to total population. About 17 percent of Sweden's 8.4 million inhabitants, or 1.4 million, are pensioners over the age of sixty-five. That proportion is expected to gradually reach the 20 percent level within the next three decades because of higher survivorship rates, better-quality care, and declining birth rates. As in other industrialized countries, the cohort of those eighty years of age and older is experiencing the most precipitous growth. Persons in this age group constituted 23 percent of all the aged in 1987, or 335,000, and they are projected to number about 450,000, or 29 percent of all the elderly, by the year 2025.

Sweden has met this demographic challenge with a remarkable array of income supports and services. They parallel, for the most part, the continuum of care found in other welfare and advanced industrial states. There is, however, a more determined public readiness to meet the needs of this aged cohort, and as a consequence, the elderly have easy access to services, most of which are extended on a nondeclining basis and without restrictive eligibility requirements.

Public Policy

Responsibility for the provision of health and social services in Sweden is shared by the three levels of government: central, regional or county, and municipal.

The parliament (*Riksdag*) sets national policies. The central administration's ministries are executive units of relatively limited operational scope. The day-to-day implementation of national policies is, instead, the domain of the more professionalized National Boards. The latter oversee the provision of services in their specific sectors and allocate government grants to counties and municipalities. Social services are thus under the political jurisdiction of the Ministry of Health and Social Affairs, but the National Board of Health and Welfare insures that policies are properly implemented. The board monitors and advises the municipal social services and ascertains that they implement programs in accordance with sanctioned legal mandates.

Sweden's twenty-three counties are each administered by a council that is responsible for health and medical care, including acute and long-term hospitalization, nursing homes, and psychiatric care. County councils levy their own taxes and operate as associations of local municipalities.

The third level of government is the municipalities. They operate the social services, recreation programs, and housing, among other programs. There are 284 such jurisdictions in Sweden, and although they enjoy a substantial measure of autonomy, they must comply with the broad policy guidelines set by the central government.

Social Services Legislation

During the early 1980s Sweden passed a series of far-reaching laws that gave new directions to the provision of health and social services. Of particular relevance for the aged and for home care are the 1982 Social Services Act and its subsequent companion, the 1983 Health and Medical Services Act.

The first, the Social Services Act (*Socialtjanstlagen*) designates most social services, including home care, as a municipal duty. The preamble to the law contains the following guiding principles:

1. *Normalization.* Individuals should be assisted to live and function in their own homes and continue leading an independent existence.

2. *Self-determination.* People have the right to make their own decisions on matters that may affect the future course of their lives.

3. *Flexibility.* Services and facilities ought to be adapted to the particular needs of each individual.

4. *Holistic perspective.* Persons' needs—social, psychological and physical—ought to be considered as a totality and placed in the context of their natural environment.

5. *Local focus.* Because people's problems are closely associated to local environmental factors, the corresponding solution or support should similarly be available in the vicinity of their homes.

The Social Services Act is a so-called "framework" law because it concerns itself, for the most part, with the rights of the individual and lays down fundamental value aspirations in the form of normative objectives. It leaves to each municipality, however, the discretion of how to design a system of services that conforms to the policy's intent. Regrettably, like most other "framework" laws, it limits itself to general principles and does not define the actual "dos and don'ts" as far as the local authorities are concerned. Because it contains few operational prescriptions, often the country's administrative courts are left to dispel ambiguities and interpret the underlying legislative intent.

The law contains two specific items directly relevant to the elderly.

The first, Article 3, stipulates that all persons are entitled not only to basic income supports but also to the services that will ensure a meaningful life and a reasonable standard of living. The article makes it clear, however, that each municipality's social welfare authority must act as the provider of last resort, and only when all other potential sources, both public and private, have been exhausted or are no longer available.

Article 6 prescribes, more specifically, that home care and home health supports must be provided for those who cannot perform independently their activities of daily living. The municipality's obligation ceases, however, if it can invoke matrimonial responsibility, that is, when it can be demonstrated that there is a relatively healthy, able-bodied spouse capable of providing at least some of the required supports.

Sweden is unique in that home care consumers may take their grievances directly to county administrative courts if they feel that their rights are being denied by the municipal social welfare authorities. Administrative courts in Sweden deal with conflicts between individuals and public agencies. An appeal may be lodged at the Administrative Appeals Court at either the regional or county level. Legal claims usually are resolved at the county level, but they may be heard by the Supreme Administrative Court if the case has no precedents and may, therefore, set new jurisprudence.

Disputes are the inevitable corollary of the absence of statutory guidelines. The 1982 act does not stipulate the volume, range, or threshold of home care services to which a person is entitled. It is up to each municipality to set its budgetary limits and service priorities. Social services consequently vary considerably from one municipality to another. Locality Y may thus prescribe five hours a week of home help, while neighboring municipality Z will provide no more than three hours to a person with similar needs. Sundstrom (1987) points to great disparities also in the overall percentage of elderly people benefiting from home help, which may range from 17 percent of those aged eighty or older to over 80 percent, depending on where one lives.

County council governments issue program guidelines aimed at establishing more uniform standards of services among municipalities but they have no authority to enforce them, and must therefore rely on a negotiated consensus with the local authorities. Administrative courts are particularly sensitive to inequities in the provision of services, yet they rarely favor the elderly plaintiff because they also take into account the budgetary constraints that afflict social welfare departments. The courts have often found that an older person's demand for more, or even twenty-four-hour services, actually reflects loneliness and feelings of anxiety rather than a real need for more home supports.

The central government's National Board of Health and Welfare regularly issues quality standards and operational guidelines for social services, medical and dental care, substance abuse, pharmaceutical services, public health, and care for the disabled, but it also respects the discretion left to the municipalities on how these services should be implemented. Municipalities must abide by those guidelines if they wish to qualify for the cost-sharing subsidy from the central government. Moreover, in the case of home care this participation has no budgetary restrictions, a departure from other government-subsidized programs such as transportation and housing. The very fact that home care is not capped clearly indicates the high priority the central government assigns to community care.

One of the distinctive features of the 1982 law is precisely the singling out of home care as a universal entitlement. Its implied intent, embodied in the already mentioned principle of "normalization," is that older persons should continue living in their own homes. It assumes that most people wish to remain in their habitual environments and, conversely, that they abhor the thought of institutional living. The new legislation consequently fosters the containment of nursing home care while favoring more home-delivered services.

In addition, national policies approve the limited provision of "service" houses or "service" flats. These are municipally owned and operated residential facilities that offer only the bare minimum of services. Residents in these apartment complexes have access to several communal facilities such as activity rooms, a lounge, a television room, and so forth. If they also need home help, the building superintendent will contact the social welfare district office. These offices may, coincidentally, be located on the very premises of the "service" houses. Home care is therefore obtained on a case-by-case basis, as an external service. It is not, however, an intrinsic service component of the residential facility.

Home care has become, without any doubt, the most commonly used of all services for the aged. For every nursing home or old age home resident in 1985, there were more than three home care users in the community (97,700 persons in institutions, as compared to a total of 320,000 recipients of home help and home health care).

However, despite this forceful promotion of the home care alternative, institutionalization rates remain high and have experienced little variation over the last twenty years. Between the years 1965 and 1975, the percentage of institutionalized elderly sixty-five years of age and older rose slightly from 7.2 percent to 8.0 percent, declining to 6.7 percent by 1985. During the same twenty-year period, consumers of home help services nearly doubled, increasing from 12.8 in 1965 to 22.8 percent in 1975, then declining to 18.8 percent in 1985 (Doyle, 1987). Thus home care does not appear to lessen the demand for nursing home care. It taps, according to Sundstrom (1985), into a different and new consumer population.

ENGLAND

The provision of health and social services in community settings rather than in institutions is a basic tenet of the British health and welfare system. With the growth of the elderly—18 percent of the population is sixty-five and over—the demand for community care has similarly expanded.

It is estimated that there are approximately one million persons over the age of sixty-five in England and Wales receiving long-term care, with the majority being cared for at home (Department of Health and Social Security, 1987). As in other industrial countries, most of the care has been provided by relatives, but as family members grow older and fewer women are available to provide complete care, the pressure for formal community care has expanded. A wide array of direct services for the elderly, which includes day care centers, respite or holiday relief, laundry services for incontinents, telephone and alarm services, physical therapy, home helps, and meals on wheels, has been developed to cope with that demand.

Public Policy on Home Care

The emphasis on community rather than institutional care for the elderly can be traced to the National Health Services Act of 1946, which assigned to local governments the discretion to make arrangements for domestic help in households where a person was ill, pregnant, mentally handicapped, or aged.

Amendments and reviews of the National Health Service completed in the 1950s emphasized the importance of community services for reducing unnecessary lengthy hospital stays by older persons. Alternative and less expensive care could be received at home. The legislative reviews stressed the need for the government to provide home-delivered meals, chiropody, and social and recreational services to support the older persons and their care givers in the community. An amendment to the National Assistance Act in 1962 encouraged local governments to provide meals, chiropody, and social and recreational programs for the elderly, although these services were to be financed locally. In order to achieve a semblance of uniformity throughout the country in the provision of these programs, the Social Services Act of 1970 delegated the task of coordinating all community services to the local social service departments.

The Health Services and Public Health Act of 1968, enacted in 1971, expanded the scope of community care by requiring that local authorities provide essential care in the home for those unable to care for themselves due to illness, childbirth, handicap, or age. In 1972 the central government ordered these authorities to submit a ten-year plan for the development of their social services along specific guidelines. One of these guidelines stipulated that there be twelve full-time home help workers per one thousand elderly.

The government's *Priorities for Health and Personal Social Services in England* (Department of Health and Social Security, 1976) emphasized the need for expanding community care by setting an increase of 3.2 percent per year as an annual goal in services for the elderly. The main objective of these services would be to help older people stay in the community as long as possible.

Subsequently, *Care in Action*—issued by the Department of Health and Social Security (1981a)—delineated the official policies and priorities for health and social services, with further emphasis on the community care needs of the frail elderly. This document underscored the service objectives but did not suggest the strategies for their implementation. The two main objectives were the following:

1. To strengthen primary and community care services as well as neighborhood and voluntary supports, so that elderly persons can continue to live at home
2. To encourage active treatment and rehabilitation of the elderly in the hospital so that they can return home

A related document, *Care in the Community*, (Department of Health and Social Security, 1981b) stressed ways in which patients and resources for their care could be transferred from the National Health Service to the personal social services in the local community. An analysis of costs spent on services showed little variation between 1974 and 1981–82 in the ratio of funds spent on hospital and community health services, with the largest proportion in each period allocated to hospital care. In 1974–75 the hospitals absorbed 63.1 percent of the health budget, while community health services received only 6.5 percent; in 1981–82 hospitals received 62.8 percent and community health services 6.7 percent (Department of Health and Social Security, 1987). Thus, although the government's policy nominally advocates community rather than institutional care, the government appears to be reluctant to allocate the proper resources to make the community programs more competitive.

The Role of the Central Government

The central government is involved in the provision of community care through the Department of Health and Social Security. The department provides grants to the 108 local authorities, 30 rural counties, and 33

London metropolitan boroughs to partially cover the costs of their social services. It also makes recommendations regarding services, but it has no authority to mandate them. Each local authority has the autonomy to distribute the funds among all of its social service programs following rough governmental guidelines.

Local authorities are obligated to plan and develop their own home care services and to deliver at least a stated minimum floor of protection. Until the early 1980s, the central government's guidelines required that each authority provide seventeen residential places, twelve home helps, and five hospital beds for every 1,000 elderly persons. Because of the differing demographic realities across the country, these guidelines have now been discarded. Instead, the government requires that each area survey its needs and develop an appropriate package of services to best meet them. The Department of Health and Social Security has developed a balance-of-care model with standards for packages of services according to levels of dependency of the population. The model, however, is intended as a framework only, and local governments are not required to follow it.

A new set of guidelines for the formulation of local policies in home care was subsequently designed by the Audit Commission for Local Authorities in England and Wales (Audit Commission, 1985). It required that policies for home care services include the following:

1. A clear statement of the aims of the service, for example, the extent of personal or domestic care
2. Explicit criteria for service, that is, their intended target groups
3. Definition of the types of clients for whom coordination with other community services might be required
4. Guidelines on frequency and length of visits
5. Guidelines for the allocation of clients to home helps
6. Procedures for allocating home help workers to geographic areas

The Social Services Inspectorate of the Department of Health and Social Security, aware of the increased significance and complexity of home care services throughout the country, decided in 1986 to assess these programs' effectiveness. This was partially in recognition of the changing roles and duties of the home helps, who were becoming more involved with personal care (Department of Health and Social Security, 1987). The initial study in 1986 focused on eight large counties in southern England, the West Midlands, and the North West, each combining both urban and rural areas. It projected that between the years 1981 and 1991 the overall population of the eight counties would increase by 4 percent. The population sixty-five and over would, however, experience a 9 percent gain, with the population seventy-five and over increasing by 22 percent. These latter demographic shifts forecast that the demand for home care services will similarly expand. If so, public policy may then have to decide whether or not to ration services through more restrictive eligibility requirements or through the allocation of resources.

All eight local authorities were unanimous in supporting the principle of home care services to assist persons to remain independent, and all had developed varying policies and structures for reaching these objectives. However, only one authority instituted priorities and criteria for services that were clearly documented. In the others, objectives were ill-defined and vague. The report concluded that although all the programs were concerned with developing policies, they had not yet reached the standards outlined by the Audit Commission. Furthermore, the study revealed varying perspectives of home care policies held by senior managers, home help organizers, and service delivery staff. In fact, direct service personnel often felt left out of policy formulation and planning and frequently had no knowledge that any formal policy even existed. As a result, one of the main recommendations of the study was that managers be involved in the design of pertinent home care policies. Finally, in order for such policies to have real effects on services, the commission outlined the following preconditions that would have to be met:

1. Strategic objectives: concrete objectives and choices

2. Budget management: procedures for constructing and allocating home help budgets that are understood and are linked to policy objectives

3. Case management frameworks: definitions of realistic and workable case management practices

4. Work structures: expectations, job descriptions, working conditions, peer group support, training, and management systems

5. Front-line management. Home help organizers need clarity about the amount of time to be allocated to case management, personnel work, budgeting, and administration while also having more reasonable work loads and being included in policy planning.

The Griffiths Report

One of the most recent governmental efforts in the community care field has been the Griffiths report, *Community Care: Agenda for Action* (Her Majesty's Stationery Office, 1988). This parliamentary document outlines a framework for policy and programs in community care and the ways in which government funds for these programs should be allocated. Some of its key recommendations are as follows:

1. Community care should be under the jurisdiction of its own Ministry.
2. Funding of social services authorities by the central government should not exceed 50 percent of their costs, in order to give primary responsibility for community care to local districts.
3. Social service authorities should make sure that needs are identified and attended to, with services coordinated under a case manager.
4. The role of the public sector is to ensure that care is provided, not necessarily to provide all the care; this may involve purchasing services from the private sector.
5. Public funding for services should be unified under one system and allocated on the basis of an individual's needs rather than through social security and local authority taxes.
6. There is the need for a new multipurpose auxiliary force of "helps" trained in the practical aspects of community care, such as assisting persons with dressing, shopping, and home cleaning.

The intent of these proposals was to reaffirm each local government's responsibility for the implementation of its community care policies while retaining control of its own fiscal resources. The proposals also reassert the participation of the private sector as care providers and the necessity to form partnerships between public and private agencies.

The initial response of Parliament to the report in the fall of 1989 recognized both the government's commitment to community care and the need to maintain persons in their own homes as long as possible. It was also recommended that a single source of funding for community care services, rather than the present separation of state and local funding, be created. The local authorities already responsible for social services would assume control of these funds and consequently for the support of persons in community, as well as for residential and nursing home care.

Local authorities, however, will not necessarily have to provide all services directly, although they will be responsible for the assessments and the care plans. In fact, as stated above, they are encouraged to use the voluntary, nonprofit and private agencies as the actual providers of services. Resources for supporting these responsibilities will be obtained by transferring to the local authorities the funds from social security that are currently used to finance care in residential and nursing homes.

Critics of these proposals are concerned about the increasing role the private sector may play in providing service. They point out that because the country has historically relied upon the public and the voluntary, nonprofit sectors, there are few regulations or licensing provisions for private agencies. New standards and means of monitoring them will have to be developed. This task alone could drain the resources of the public sector.

Although the government professes a commitment to community care, its actions are not consistent with its stated objectives. It continues to support persons who are financially eligible in residential homes at the rate of £130 a week, while making no comparable allocation to persons receiving home care. The eventual adoption of the Griffiths report recommendations could alter this through a unified budget which would support people in either institutions or their own homes.

THE NETHERLANDS

The Netherlands has a population of 14 million, 12 percent of which is composed of persons over the age of sixty-five. This proportion is expected to increase to 15 percent by the year 2000 (Kastelein and Schouten, 1986). The majority of these older persons live at home independently, without assistance. However, approximately 12 percent of the elderly reside in residential care facilities and nursing homes, while another 10 percent, primarily those persons aged seventy-five and older, receive formal care at home (Linzel, 1986). Among those eighty and over, 16 percent receive home help services while 7.6 percent benefit from home nursing. (Klassen–Van der Berg, 1985).

Public Policy

The Netherlands consists of twelve provinces. These, in turn, comprise seven hundred municipalities which are responsible for the administration and provision of health and welfare services. Most of these services, including home help, home nursing, and homes for the aged, are operated by independent, nonprofit local or district organizations that are subsidized directly by the government and through a national insurance system. Those organizations have national offices that coordinate policy development, lobby with the state legislature, and promote educational activities.

The social service system is made up of three primary sectors: social security, social welfare, and health care. Each has developed separately and to a large extent continues to function independently, often leading to an overlap and duplication of services. Policies on the elderly are administered by the ministries of Employment and Social Security; Housing; Planning and Environment; and Welfare, Health, and Cultural Affairs. The latter has established a steering committee on the care of the elderly whose aim is to coordinate national policies. It must be noted, however, that this committee's role is to advise, finance, and stimulate the nonprofit organizations that are the actual implementers of the programs for the elderly.

The government's first move toward instituting a more cohesive system of care for the elderly began in the 1960s, when it focused on the establishment of care homes for those elderly requiring assistance in meeting daily needs. This policy resulted in the Netherlands developing a large number of residential care facilities, congregate housing, sheltered housing, and apartment houses with special services. Approximately 10 percent of the older population lives in these special housing units, while another 2 percent reside in nursing homes (Kastelein and Schouten, 1986).

As of the 1970s, the initial policy toward institutionalization began to shift to a focus on community care. The increasing numbers of elderly persons, the costs of residential care, and the desire of most older persons to remain independent in their own homes provided the legitimation for this change in policy. Since the 1980s, the government's emphasis has been on increasing the coordination of the home care providers, general practitioners, social workers, home nurses, and home helps while also raising the standards of quality of care. It is important also to note that health care includes the social services and is not restricted to a medical definition.

The government is currently stressing a policy of "substitution" of services. This is defined as the systematic replacement of costly services with less expensive ones (Committee on Health Care Structure and Financing, 1987). It involves not only adopting home care as a substitute for institutional care, but also fostering informal supports in place of formal services whenever feasible.

A governmental steering group to study the future of health services was formed in 1983. The group produced a report that outlined three possible scenarios, as follows:

1. The "reference" scenario—demographic changes will result in an increased demand for care.

2. The "growth" scenario—there will be mounting pressure to expand the care system, given the elderlies' expectations of receiving more services.

3. The "shrinkage" scenario—changing attitudes in society will encourage persons to care for themselves and to pay attention to primary prevention. This will ultimately result in improved general health status and a lower need for services.

A 1989 evaluation of these scenarios found that greater numbers of elderly persons are remaining in their own homes, although there has not been a concomitant increase in domiciliary services (Kastelein, Dijkstra, and Schouten, 1989). The gap in services appears to have been filled by volunteer programs. There is no evidence that the "shrinkage" scenario has begun to take effect.

The government in the Netherlands had initially fostered the development of professional services, but since the early 1980s it has voiced increasing interest in promoting informal care givers. However, there has been little actual allocation of funds to support these informal care systems. Furthermore, instituting such a policy would be questionable, given that legislation has already affirmed the right to "optimal" services, meaning professional care. In fact, the elderly seem to prefer professional to informal or familial assistance. It is also feared that a policy that would reduce professional services without concomitant additional support for care givers could stress these informal systems. To date, there has been no move to offer financial support or payments to these care givers.

The professional care system is made up of three systems: (1) social security, (2) social care that provides nonmedical community care, and (3) health care that includes medical care in the community as well as residential care.

Most social welfare services are under the authority of the national Department of Welfare, Health, and Cultural Affairs, but the ongoing administration is conducted by the local governments and the services themselves. Resources to support the services come from general taxes. Unlike the other two professional-care systems, there is very little formal legislation governing social care. It tends to be controlled by governmental regulations that are formulated by administrative departments rather than through parliamentary decisions. This distinction means that these programs are more vulnerable to policy shifts and budget cuts (Kastelein, Dijkstra, and Schouten, 1989).

Historically, the social care services evolved from religious and charitable organizations. The programs have tended to remain fragmented and to function autonomously without any real coordination. However, recently there has been visible governmental pressure for agencies that provide similar or overlapping services to merge into larger organizations.

The health care system consists of three organizational levels: basic health care, primary health care, and secondary health care. The basic health services are also controlled by municipal administrations and include health planning and epidemiological research. Primary health care services are those provided by general practitioners, midwives, and district nurses, while the secondary health care level clusters the medical specializations and their corresponding services.

MANITOBA, CANADA

Canada, and the United States share, in addition to a common border, many other characteristics. Both have a similar age distribution, their elderly populations are growing at a similar rate, and those over the age of eighty-five years are increasing in numbers at a faster rate. Canada, like the United States, has a federal system of government, with both the federal and lower-level (in this case provincial) governments raising and allocating revenues.

The country is divided into ten provinces that, since the late 1960s, have offered a universal health care program to all citizens. Within this system, several of the provinces have extended the coverage to include long-term care services. The province of Manitoba has developed one of the most extensive of these programs, as it integrates and coordinates both nursing home and home care into a single framework. Manitoba's publicly funded long-term care program is the oldest in the country, and home care is a critical part of this service.

Manitoba has a population of over 1 million, mostly concentrated in Winnipeg and other urban centers. A smaller proportion is distributed throughout the province's 240,000 square miles. The population aged sixty-five and over constitutes approximately 12 percent of the population, with those eighty-five and over constituting 20 percent of the aged (Manitoba Health Services Commission, 1987). To meet the needs of this older population, the province has developed a well-planned and structured system of home care services that strives to maintain persons in their own homes, at the highest possible level of independent functioning.

National Policy towards Home Care

The Canadian government has not adopted an official policy on home care but has left the initiative for enactment and implementation to the provinces. Home care is not included in the federal Medical Care and Hospital Care Act. To date, health legislation in Canada has primarily centered on overall medical and hospital acute care.

Although the Department of National Health and Welfare established a committee for developing pilot home care programs in 1957, it was not until the 1970s that home care programs began emerging throughout the country (Chappell, 1985). It was also during this period that Canada made a national reappraisal of the provinces' health care delivery system.

Canadians had been accustomed to universally insured hospital and medical services that required little or no contribution or payment on the part of the individual. Most beneficiaries were thus covered for short-term home care delivered primarily under the auspices of a hospital. On the other hand, long-term community care, the type needed most by the elderly, was not an insured entitlement. Thus those who required this type of care had no alternative but to purchase it on a private basis.

Following the health system reappraisal, home care was finally acknowledged as a service in its own right, and social services were viewed as a necessary part of the program. The federal government established, thereafter, a series of broad guidelines for home care.

> Home care should be regarded as a basic mode of health care that coordinates and/or provides the variety of personal health and supportive services required to maintain or to help function adequately in the home, those persons with health and/or social needs related to physical or mental disability, personal or family crises or to illness of an acute or chronic nature. A prerequisite is that the home is judged to be a viable place where treatment or care can be provided. Supportive services include social services and other services to assist such persons and their families. (National Health and Welfare, 1975)

Funding for home care is covered by two primary federal sources: the Established Program Financing Act, which provides for the health aspects of home care, and the Canada Assistance Plan.

The Canada Assistance Plan funds home support programs such as homemakers and other social service programs. Costs for social care are shared on a 50/50 matching basis with the provinces. The budgets of these two programs provide for most home care services, although the provinces may further supplement these funds from other provincial sources. In some provinces additional funds for home care are collected through users' fees for services.

The provinces may decide independently what services to provide under the assistance plan and how much to allocate to each. The federal government does provide minimal support for staff and guidelines to the provinces regarding expenditures. It will also share the cost of evaluations of programs with the provinces under the Canada Assistance Plan. Barriers occur, however, in sharing program ideas across provinces or in encouraging their adaptations, due to differing political orientations and philosophies.

Home Care in Manitoba

An early study on the needs of the elderly, *Aging in Manitoba* (Manitoba Department of Health and Social Development, 1973) found that community services for this population were often inaccessible or unavailable, thus resulting in the unnecessary institutionalization of a large proportion of older persons (Ewanchyna, Collins, and Block, 1980). Many elderly were forced to remain in the hospital because essential services could not be provided at home. This provincial investigation uncovered problems of fragmentation, waste, and inefficiency. The findings resulted in recommendations for a comprehensive home care program.

The Manitoba Continuing Care Program was thus initiated in 1974, in part as a response to the national evaluation of the health services. The original plan, *A Home Care Program for Manitoba* (Government of Manitoba, 1974), recommended that the service be decentralized and placed under its own administration rather than under the more generic administration of health services. This led to the establishment of a central office that coordinates home care services into an integrated program for the entire province.

The Value Premises

The underlying philosophy of Manitoba's continuing care program is that home care is preferable to institutional care and that it plays an essential role in its own right within the continuum of long-term care services. Nursing homes are viewed as an extension of home care or as the required step in those instances when home care services are no longer effective or when the capacity for community care is exhausted.

Home care in Manitoba is, consequently, seen as an alternative to nursing home placement and as a means of avoiding institutionalization. The program developed out of a need to reduce both costs and fragmentation of services. Under the Long-Term Care Insurance Act of 1973, home care was given equal status to the other health services. All persons are legally entitled to this social insurance and thus to home care, which is comparable to care in hospitals or nursing homes. In fact, patients may remain in the hospital while waiting for nursing home placements only if their care needs cannot be safely attended to in the home.

The home care program is defined more as a "support" than a "primary care program." This definition limits the program's parameters because it presumes that there is a responsible person in the client's network who takes the lead in providing assistance, or who can be called upon to do so. The home care program is not intended to provide total care.

The value principles underlying Manitoba's policy on home care are: (1) home care must be consistent with a cultural tradition which values home and family; (2) it must help the family and informal supports to cope with illness and disability; (3) it must link health and social services; (4) it must acknowledge the role of the community in a person's life; (5) it must promote the use of appropriate services; (6) it must enhance the continuity of care; and (7) it must guarantee universal access regardless of ability to pay, age, or type or duration of disability (Havens, 1987a).

In order to implement these principles most effectively, home care operates under the Office of Continuing Care, which is a part of the provincial Ministry of Health. The Office, located in Winnipeg, is responsible for the planning and programming of policy and services in home care for Manitoba's ten administrative regions. In this planning role, the Office is also responsible for the system's budgeting, program evaluation, and monitoring. Basic to the home care program are provisions for case coordination, health and social assessments, and personal supervision.

The Regional Structure of Home Care

Each of the ten regions has a continuing-care coordinator responsible for the planning, development, organization, and coordination of the Continuing Care Program. These professionals supervise the case coordinators, who make individual assessments, develop personalized care plans, and ensure the delivery of services. The case coordinators are either nurses or social workers and, depending on the region, they may work in teams. The regional continuing-care coordinators also supervise the resource developers, who are responsible for the recruitment, placement, and supervision of the home care workers. The provincial Office of Continuing Care funds the regional home care programs, but these regional programs often do not receive their requested levels of appropriations. As a consequence, regional offices frequently overspend their budgets, especially since the only restrictions on home care are that the expenditures do not exceed the equivalent level of institutional costs. Moreover, programs are mandated to offer care consistent with the client's assessed needs. Thus, if a region exhausts its budget and still has remaining unattended cases, it can continue to provide care in the expectation that the provincial government will ultimately cover the deficit. To rectify this, it has been suggested that regions be allocated fixed budgets for home care and not be provided with any supplements until reviewed and approved by the Office of Continuing Care.

ARGENTINA

Argentina shares many of the cultural, demographic, and social policy features found in the more industrialized and advanced Western societies. A low and declining birth rate coupled with a relatively high life expectancy has led to the same overrepresentation of the aged in its total population. The proportion of the cohort of those sixty years of age and older approaches the 13 percent level, but it is actually closer to 20 percent in many of the larger urban centers. In the capital city of Buenos Aires, which contains almost one-third of the country's 28 million people, 22 percent of the population is sixty years of age or older. Between 1950 and 1980 the city's proportion of aged rose from 76 percent, while in the whole country it increased from 7.04 to 12.41 percent. It is anticipated that the population of those sixty and over will surpass the 15 percent level by the year 2025.

Contrary to what is observed in many other developing countries, most of the Argentine elderly, 86.7 percent, live in urban areas where health care and formal services are more readily available. Urbanization has, however, contributed to weakening the traditional pattern of multigenerational households still prevalent in the rural areas. Public policy underscores family responsibility in the care of the aged, but many elderly feel isolated and unsupported. The rural aged are no exception. They tend to be left behind by their children when the latter join the relentless exodus of the young seeking better-paying industrial and service jobs in the major urban centers.

Public Policy

Argentina was one of the first countries of the world to foster "aging"-specific legislation. The 1949 amendments to the national constitution included a bill of "aging" rights, called the "decalogue," or ten commandments of the aged. They referred to the rights to housing, food, dress, leisure, work, peacefulness, respect, physical and mental health care, and income maintenance. The statement of rights had been previously advanced by the Eva Perón Foundation, created by President Juan D. Perón's wife. Almost simultaneously Argentina placed the same bill of rights on the United Nations agenda. It was adopted by the Third General Assembly in December 1948. This was the first time that this international forum became formally aware of the realities and needs of the elderly.

Public policy in Argentina does not envisage the care or support of the aged, however, outside the realm of the family. The foremost policy priority is, therefore, to strengthen the family unit. In its 1982 Document submitted to the United Nations World Assembly on the Aging, the Argentine government emphatically affirmed that the aged should be cared for by their relatives and should continue living in their natural communities. Public services are acknowledged as a legitimate intervention only when the family no longer exists or is no longer capable of assisting its frail older members (Ministerio de Acción Social, 1982).

Home care services are subsumed under the comprehensive national system of health care for the aged, which dates back to 1971. This system is administered by the Ministry of Social Action through its National Institute of Social Services for Retirees and Pensioners and, more directly, by its Comprehensive Medical Care Program, known by its acronym PAMI (*Programa de Atención Médica Integral*). It covers all persons sixty years of age and older who are eligible by virtue of their past work-related contributions to the social security system or related public pension programs. Eligibility alone does not guarantee access to services, however. Potential beneficiaries must register with PAMI to that effect. It is on the basis that this program serves about 3 million registered contributors to social security.

Financing and Allocation of Resources

As stated, the Argentine home health care program is part of the national health services. The latter is financed by a specially earmarked social security tax of 3 percent on all wages. The Instituto Nacional also receives funds from taxes on legalized gambling and horse races. Retirees are entitled to all medical services free of charge—dentistry included—provided they accumulate the necessary credits based on past contributions. Entitlement to services, however, is not granted automatically after retirement. Potential users must register to that effect in their corresponding institute's local district office. As mentioned earlier, the PAMI system has approximately 3 million registrants, 1.4 million of whom—almost half—reside in the *conurbano*, that is, the capital city of Buenos Aires and its surroundings. They are attended by twenty-five hundred primary physicians directly contracted by PAMI. The system, at least nominally, operates as a true national health insurance program.

Despite its deliberate centralization and administrative uniformity, the PAMI system allows for some latitude in the interpretation and implementation of nationally set statutes and regulations. Some chiefs of the twenty-nine regional delegations—properly designated as *delegados*—follow those statutes to the letter. Others are more daring and make decisions on their own when no rules or precedents are at hand to assist them. They may decide, among other things, on the apportionment of resources for home care.

These decisions may be contingent on a series of regional factors. To begin with, there is a more pronounced sense of family responsibility and consequently a lower demand for home care services in the rural provinces or districts. Also and as already mentioned, districts in the *conurbano*, those in the Buenos Aires greater metropolitan area, do their own contracting of participating primary physicians. District chiefs here make their own determination of how many physicians are needed based on demographics, indicators of need, and resources available.

Delegations in the interior, that is, the rest of the country beyond the greater Buenos Aires metropolitan area, do not enjoy the same discretionary power. They can no longer purchase services from individual physicians, but must proceed instead through the provincial medical associations, which act as intermediaries. This third-party arrangement was instituted for reasons of administrative expediency: PAMI wished to avoid the administrative chores of recruiting, monitoring, and compensating each individual physician. The provincial medical associations assume all these tasks and also institute and enforce quality-of-care standards. In exchange for all this, they collect an indirect cost rate, which is deducted from the physicians' compensations. The medical associations thus obtain both a substantial overhead from the country's health care bill and the power to farm out the assignments or quotas of registered elderly to their own members. Physicians wishing to supplement their income with these PAMI quotas of eligible elderly have no alternative but to join their local medical association and accept its contractual terms.

CONCLUSION

The countries studied adhere to policies that stress home rather than institutional care. Increasing numbers of older persons and rising costs of services, combined with the recognition that most older persons want to stay in their own homes, have contributed to this policy orientation. Some countries began with the liberal promotion of institutional services but then changed towards promotion of community-based home care. There is, however, substantial variation concerning the roles reserved to their national and local governments with regard to the planning and administration of long-term care services. Some tend to operate such services in a tightly centralized fashion through federal or provincial agencies assigning minimal discretion to state or local governments. In such instances, services respond to standard guidelines and controls, having little room for local initiatives.

Other countries adopt a decentralized system whereby local and municipal jurisdictions are allowed to shape their own programs, consistent with local needs, idiosyncracies and traditions. Central governments in such cases promulgate broad normative guidelines, only defining the floor of services that must be made available. This is a minimalist framework, beyond which local governments enjoy substantial flexibility and self-determination. Decentralization is therefore intended to encourage local innovation and community initiative. Centralization is, in turn, praised because it seemingly insures greater equity in access to services.

4

The Organization and Operation of Home Care Services

This chapter describes and analyzes the organization, operation, and financing of home care in each of the six countries. Particular consideration is given to the coordination of services with other health and community services, the range of variations in administrative approaches, and, finally, how the services actually reach their intended beneficiaries.

NORWAY

Types of Service

Home care consists of two specific services: home help and home nursing. The first is by far the most extensive service with respect to the number of persons it reaches and benefits. Its aim is to assist those frail elderly and disabled who would otherwise be unable to continue living independently. The home help service includes light housework, shopping, laundry, meals preparation, window washing, and related daily tasks. Although home help is not restricted to the elderly, they are the primary users of the service.

Home nursing is the fastest-growing form of home help and serves as a viable alternative to institutionalization for those elderly who can manage with less intensive medical care and/or supervision. The types of services available through the home nursing program are information and counseling, curative treatment, rehabilitation, and general nursing care. As with home help, home nursing is not age-specific, but most patients for this service as well are over the age of sixty-five. The total number of home nursing patients in 1985 was 52,258, of whom 79 percent were aged sixty-seven and older. Home help clients in 1984 numbered 112,196, with 87 percent being sixty-seven years of age or older.

Overall, 10.2 percent of the population between the ages of sixty-seven and seventy-nine and 26.9 percent of those aged eighty years and older benefit from home nursing services. Yet variations from county to county are staggering. Only 13.2 percent of the octogenarians in Oslo, as opposed to 42.5 in More and Romsdal, receive home nursing care.

Costs and Distribution of Services

Charges for home help services are established on a sliding scale basis. In 1982, service charges to individuals covered about 7 percent of the gross costs of home help services. The bulk of the cost is defrayed by municipalities. Home nursing, on the other hand, as of 1984 has been free of charge for all patients. Since 1989 every municipality in Norway has provided home help and nearly all have offered home nursing services.

The total number of units of home nursing care services for the entire country during 1986 was 6,361,312, an increase of 10.4 percent over the preceding year. This can be translated into an average of 60.1 units or visits per actual consumer, although the range is, once again, quite broad, from 38.9 visits for More and Romsdal county to 81.7 for Vestfold county.

As established in the Social Care Act, community services for the aged are under the authority of the municipalities. As of January, 1988, both old age homes and nursing homes have fallen under municipal jurisdiction. The counties, in turn, are responsible for hospital care and psychiatric nursing home care services. The costs of the latter are covered by the counties' own budgets as well as state block grants and National Health Insurance funds. Assistance is provided on a nondeclining basis, regardless of personal income or assets.

The Ministry of Health and Social Affairs assumes 50 percent of the nursing home costs and 75 percent of the expenses connected with home nursing (the remainder of each is covered by the municipalities). While the Ministry of Health subsidizes municipal home help programs, the Ministry of Labor and Local Governments supports the provision of housing for the elderly.

In principle, each municipality's social welfare board operates the home help services unless this function has been delegated to a special committee or other specialized agency. The social welfare board's responsibilities include supervision of activities; coordination with other governmental committees, health authorities, and private organizations; assessments of need for service; development of new assessment measures; and refinement of existing service arrangements. The municipalities retain the discretion to organize the delivery of services in a way that best fits their overall policy priorities (Guntvedt, 1985).

It is not surprising, therefore, that the organization of home help varies from municipality to municipality. In practice, the director of home nursing in each of these local authorities attends the day-to-day management of both the home helper services and the home nursing service. The ultimate authority delegated to each municipality is further broken down at the district level. Oslo has recently embarked in a major decentralization drive, entailing the city's division into twenty-five relatively autonomous districts.

The initial steps in the implementation of the above model have been rather difficult. Professional nurses, for instance, resist going into the community. Consequently, home helpers may have to expand their habitual tasks and take on more of the basic responsibilities currently performed by nurse's aides. As a result, the distinction between the two may eventually narrow, although it will not necessarily disappear.

One of the major objectives of the new move toward decentralization has been to allocate smaller clusters of workers for each district. These workers may have different occupational backgrounds, but they are expected to operate in team fashion. The main obstacle is that most of these workers lack experience or adequate preparation to work in such team arrangements.

A goal of decentralization is that it will enhance equity and equal access to services. However, it remains doubtful that this equality can truly be attained. For three years Oslo experimented with decentralization in four of the twenty-five districts into which it will be divided. The evaluation revealed that needy, low-income persons who never used services still did not avail themselves of the programs. The more educated and economically advantaged continued to be the ones who maximized the use of public services.

Oslo: A Case Example of Decentralization

Prior to the implementation of the decentralization policies, Oslo was divided into fourteen service districts. A site visit and interviews with the staff of District 2, Slemdalsveien, provided insight into the daily operations of the municipal home care service network.

The district is divided into four subdistricts, each with its own budget and a relatively high degree of autonomy. Each of the four subdistricts includes three layers of administrative authority. The first is an overall administrator. Immediately underneath is a chief for health and social services. The third level, in turn, includes the sections responsible for home nursing, home help, nursing home care, and congregate housing. Subdistricts may buy or lend services from each other during peak activity periods. A head nurse is assigned to each subdistrict, assisted by several nurse's aides and at least one occupational therapist, one physical therapist, and a podiatrist.

There are two or three home nursing teams in each subdistrict. Each team carries a caseload of forty to fifty patients and is staffed by two registered nurses and three to four nurse's aides. This work-load apportionment is based on a population formula that takes into account the number of persons over age seventy, the number of children below age 15 (which includes a large number of children of immigrants and refugees), and the social conditions prevalent in the area. Budgetary allocations, including the number of nursing home beds, are contingent on these factors. A source of major concern has been that while the number of patients requesting home care services has remained constant, both the intensity and frequency of needed services have increased dramatically. This is due to the fact that these patients constitute an older, more chronically handicapped population.

Full-time home nursing workers rarely see more than three clients in the course of a 7½-hour day. Services range from a minimum of a half hour to three hours per client per day. The average is three hours per client per week, and may not exceed ten weekly hours. If clients need more assistance, they will be referred to institutional care.

Home help workers are organized into teams with a maximum of fifteen workers, each led by a group leader. The district leader assumes the responsibility for conducting the first visit to all new applicants. This is done no later than two weeks after receiving the request for services. Self-referrals are accepted, but requests for services originate for the most part in hospitals or outpatient clinics. After the initial home visit by the district leader, a tentative assessment is completed and a service plan is made. The rate of denials is rather minimal. In the case of District 2, there were no more than twenty such rejections in the preceding four-year period. Moreover, people do not abuse the system, since they do not want to admit that they need help. Home care is stigmatizing, as it is equated in the public mind with dependency.

The district leader assigns special importance to the initial interview. The assessment revolves around four central questions:

1. What can you do for yourself?
2. What can't you do?
3. Do you have anybody else to help you?

4. What can we do for you? (Asked if the answer to Question 3 is affirmative.)

In the infrequent cases when the evaluation or the prognosis is inconclusive, the district leader will request that the home health nurse and/or the district physician make an additional visit. The home health nurses, by and large, are familiar with each case and tend to be more restrictive in the prescription of home care services.

Referrals, Assessments, and Service Provision

Throughout the country, district offices may negotiate with a referring hospital to keep a patient a few extra days until a home nurse can be assigned to the case. The discharging hospital can recommend a specific service, but the ultimate decision rests in the hands of each municipality's social welfare board.

District head nurses decide the length of home care services for each patient. However, this is tentative, and each individual's condition ultimately determines how much service is required. Patients are visited by home nurses an average of three times a week, yet a sizable number are seen on a daily basis. Most visits are conducted in the morning hours, but the number of evening visits is increasing due to the higher levels of disability of the population under care. Each visit lasts between thirty minutes and two hours. It may be limited to administering medication, but it may also include attending to the person's emotional concerns.

Social workers are seldom brought in to assume these tasks. They handle, instead, discrete assignments such as entitlements and financial planning, requests for protective services, and the initiation of procedures for declarations of incompetence. There is, however, no standardization of the methods for the provision of home nursing or home help, and many municipalities have been experimenting with service models that better fit their needs and conditions.

SWEDEN

Definition of Home Care Services

Home care, usually called "noninstitutional" or "open" old age care (Sundstrom, 1987), actually consists of three categories of services: home help, home health, and heavy-duty cleaning, although this is considered a separate component of home help.

Home help has emerged over the years as the most frequently consumed service among the aged. In 1985 it was utilized by almost 20 percent of the population sixty-five years of age and older, and by 44 percent of those over age eighty. This represented some 320,000 beneficiaries, who were assisted by some 76,000 home helpers, who in turn were monitored by 2,700 supervisors. Moreover, home care has been growing at an 8 percent annual rate, in terms of needed full-time manpower inputs (The Swedish Institute, 1988).

The capital city of Stockholm offers a wide array of home help services that include assistance with dressing and personal care, reminders to take medications, garbage removal, shopping, cooking and delivery meals from service centers' kitchens, housecleaning, weekly laundry, care of clothing, errands to banks and post offices, socialization, walks, and escorting. The home help staff is not expected, however, to provide heavy-duty cleaning such as washing windows, curtains, and walls, and so forth. These tasks are performed by separate teams that confine themselves exclusively to home maintenance, not interacting with the resident. This service, however, makes up only a small portion of the total hours of service provided by the home help system.

Financing Home Care Services for the Aged

Municipalities receive a state subsidy but must rely for the most part on their own tax levies to finance their budgeted expenditures. Nearly two-thirds of all services for the aged are covered through municipal taxes. The central government contributes about 20 percent, while the balance, or approximately 15 percent, is derived from patients' fees. Disaggregating the central state's participation by municipal categories of geriatric services reveals that home help is subsidized at the 30 percent level. Most local authorities charge for home help on a sliding scale based on personal income. But they barely recover 7 percent of the total costs. Municipal charges for home help are not uniform even within the same income levels, but vary according to frequency of use. The most dependent and severely handicapped, who require more than twenty-five hours of service a week, are charged proportionally less than those who are infrequent users, but there are staggering regional variations in the corresponding rates. Unlike home help, home health care is totally free and is disbursed from counties' budgets.

Services for the aged tend to be a dominant category in municipal budgets. In the case of Jönkoping, a city of 300,000, 35.5 percent of the net municipal expenses for social services were allocated to the aged in 1988. This constituted about 11 percent of the total municipal budget. Expenses for the aged were followed closely by amounts allocated to services for children, which received 32.6 percent. All remaining services and administrative operations absorbed the balance, or slightly less than one-third of the budget. Housing allowances received 12.2 percent, income supplements 8.7 percent, administration 6.7 percent, and alcoholism and substance abuse 4.3 percent.

Organization of Services

Municipalities are rather free to experiment and test different modalities of service once they comply with the basic requirements set by the central government. Most have created extensive round-the-clock systems of home care. A typical municipal government is divided, for service delivery purposes, into districts. There are eighteen such districts in the capital city and five in a relatively medium-sized city like Jönkoping. Each district's office of social services is headed by a manager who reports to the city's director of social services. The district managers oversee several branch—or subdistrict—managers. They, in turn, have command over the subdistrict supervisors, who come in direct contact with the home help workers. The latter, finally, are organized in teams, each coordinated by one of the home help workers themselves. Each subdistrict supervisor oversees an average of twenty-eight home helpers and is responsible for about 120 active cases.

This five-step ladder may seem excessively bureaucratized, but it was designed to bring services as close and as fast as possible to their target population. Each subdistrict cares for some two hundred elderly service consumers, and its offices are easily accessible in the community. Home helpers can similarly reach any of their clients from their base office in a matter of minutes, if not seconds.

Home help services must be offered on a nondeclining basis commensurate to an individual's needs. Because of the strong belief that people should remain in their natural environment, there is no threshold beyond which it may be decided that institutionalization is a preferable and more cost-effective course of action.

County governments have been reducing the number of nursing home beds in a move aimed at ultimately dismantling all forms of institutional care. The immediate effect of this policy has been to exacerbate the demand for home help, including night care, a responsibility that municipalities must also bear. It is not surprising, therefore, that local governments complain that the counties' strategy amounts to a virtual transfer of fiscal obligations. They accuse the counties of cutting services and placing the burden of unattended needs on the localities, for which the latter get no additional budgetary relief. The counties counterargue that their nursing homes are populated by older and sicker persons whose care is becoming increasingly more intensive and costly.

Home Health Care

Home health care or home nursing care is the second major category of home care and is delivered for the most part by visiting nurses, usually based in a county council's primary-care offices.

A typical county may be divided into three or four major health districts which, in turn, comprise several primary-care subdistrict offices that are easily accessible to the residents in the area. Each of these primary-care offices is staffed with physicians, nurses, and occupational and physical therapists. In addition, these offices operate transitional or group living facilities. In Jönkoping county, each subdistrict has also at least one special group living unit for six to eight demented residents in an ordinary apartment building. Given the high demand for such facilities, the county council aims to develop a total of twenty-five units by 1992. This objective is still inadequate to meet the estimated need.

In Jönkoping the provision of home health services usually starts with a referral made by a hospital's attending nurse prior to a patient's discharge. The subdistrict head nurse will initiate the assessment, often teaming up with the municipal home help subdistrict supervisor, and occasionally also in consultation with the subdistrict's primary-care physician. The parties will arrive at a service plan and review it jointly at stipulated intervals. The head nurse, usually a licensed registered nurse, supervises the home visiting nurses who will implement the service plan. They are for the most part nurse's aides attached to either day or night services. A typical day starts at 8 A.M. with a review of the reports of the "night patrol" for the preceding night. The telephone begins ringing at the same time that patients make requests. Between 9 A.M. and 4:30 P.M. the nurses are in the field visiting up to twelve patients each. Rarely do they visit fewer than five in a single day. The "night patrol" arrives at 4:30 P.M., relieving the daytime workers. Each subdistrict has at least one "night patrol" operating in two shifts: 6:00 to 9:00 P.M. and 9:00 P.M. to 6:00 A.M. Visiting nurses carefully avoid performing home help tasks and sometimes even delegate some nursing services, such as changing wound dressings and administering insulin injections, to the home help worker.

According to Zatterqvist (1987), most of the home health care recipients in Jönkoping—77.5 percent—have chronic conditions that require indefinite care. Many have lived in nursing homes, while others manage to avoid institutionalization because of the availability of this service. Patients requiring short-term posthospital rehabilitation constitute approximately 14 percent of the caseload, while terminal patients requiring 24-hour home care make up less than 1 percent (.9 percent). The balance, 7.5 percent, are acute care cases.

Home health care proves to be for the most part cheaper than nursing home care. This was the case with 76.3 percent of the recipients in Jön-koping in 1986. In 21.2 percent of the cases home care fell below the costs of a skilled-level facility but exceeded those of a less intensive level of institutional care. Home care was more expensive than intensive nursing home care for only 2.5 percent of the cases. A typical example of the latter was a 102-year-old man living alone and receiving the services of both a home helper and a home health nurse four times a day, seven days a week (Zatterqvist, 1987).

There is no limit to the home nursing services a sick or convalescent person may receive. It is not inconceivable that terminally ill persons may require round-the-clock attention if they choose to die at home. County councils aim to respect this wish but cannot always fully comply with it.

The Service House Concept

Home care is frequently dispensed in the previously mentioned municipal service houses, that is, residential facilities that combine private apartments with congregate dining and limited recreational programming. Home care is available on a case-by-case basis but is not part of the building's own administered services. It is instead a part of the overall municipal home care system and is brought in to meet the needs of any eligible resident.

Because policymakers abhor the medical model inherent in long-stay facilities, these service houses are conceived as a form of independent living, with services added only on an ad hoc basis. There is a nutrition program that usually operates on the main floor, with a cafeteria open to the aged from the surrounding neighborhood. This program also prepares and acts as a distribution center of meals for the shut-in and disabled older persons living alone in the community. Their home helpers collect these meals.

Community elderly may also participate in the recreational day or socialization programs. The main floor is thus a virtual senior drop-in center and is the central station for all the "lifeline" alarms of the community elderly. If calls occur at night, the service house staff will alert the "night patrol" of home helpers. They in turn, contact the watchmen of a private security company contracted to keep the keys to all "lifeliners'" apartments. A watchman is then dispatched together with a district home help worker to check on the probable emergency.

Social planners meticulously seek to advance and sustain a social model of independent living, but the needs of the residents, as well as the expectations voiced by their families and hospital discharge staff, often clash with this intent. Most service house residents are very advanced in age. Many are also single. A substantial number are confused and incapable of making appropriate personal decisions. They consequently require protective services, and their needs exceed the range of services available on the premises. Relatives often voice their disappointment over the lack of more custodial attention. They would like to assume that the facility is in reality a nursing home, and cannot understand the distinction of service objectives.

It is not surprising, therefore, that home help is used almost universally by service house residents, as was the case with eighty-three of the ninety residents in Jönkoping's Tarpa House. For practical reasons, the municipal department of social welfare has installed a subdistrict office on Tarpa's premises to attend both internal and community calls for home help service. Its teams of home helpers combine both service house and community residents in the daily schedules, but the service requirements of the former tend to be far more intensive and time consuming. However, given that placements in more intensive settings are almost unavailable, service houses have turned into the permanent residences for a rather heterogeneous population, ranging from moderate to severe levels of frailty. With the aging of the residents, the likelihood of further deterioration will increase, thus compounding the prospective intensification of their dependency needs. It is questionable whether service houses will then be able to retain the appearance of independent living.

ENGLAND

From Home Help to Personal Home Care

Home help constitutes the dominant form of community care. Thirty percent of the total social services budget for the elderly goes for home help. Conversely, 65 percent of the elderly receiving general social services also receive home help (Department of Health and Social Security, 1987). The proportion of the elderly receiving home help services varies, however, by location. In some areas the service is targeted on those most in need, while in others it is spread over as many beneficiaries as possible.

Home help has been a part of every local authority since 1948 (National Council on Home Help Services, 1979). Beginning as an independent service, the home help programs have since been incorporated into the local social services departments, where they compete with residential care for the limited municipal funds.

Home help started as a domiciliary service, but as clients have become older and frailer, it has progressively introduced more elements of personal care. During the eighties, this has resulted in a transition to home care, since it has extended beyond the original domestic duties while also expanding to meet the reality that clients' needs cannot always be met between the hours of 9 A.M. and 5 P.M. Thus some local authorities have assigned workers to twenty-four-hour shifts. In some instances, a worker may even live with a client for a short period of time. This gradual transition to personal home care is occurring throughout the country. An outcome has been the enhanced status of home help workers, since they are now considered personal care givers rather than domestic helps.

A useful classification of home help services developed by Dexter and Harbert (1983) includes the following:

1. Tending
    A. The living environment—assistance in carrying out duties necessary to maintain the cleanliness, safety, and security of the home
    B. Food—shopping, preparing, and cooking if necessary
    C. Warmth—cleaning grates, lighting fires, tending heaters
    D. Personal care—helping the client in and out of bed, dressing and undressing, and attending to personal cleanliness
2. Rehabilitation
    A. Health—motivating clients to maintain therapy set by medical and nursing services
    B. Household management—teaching and advising on nutrition, cooking, budgeting
    C. Control—assuming direct family responsibilities in relation to income and expenditure

Organization of Home Help Programs

Home help services are not uniformly organized throughout the country. Their only commonality is that they are located within departments of social services. Three basic models of management have been identified (Rowbottom, Hey, and Billis, 1978).

1. Outposting, in which the service is headed by an administrator based in the central social services department with management responsibility for all direct services provided through local offices.
2. Attachment, in which overall administrative control is retained in the central office, but daily operational control of activities is exercised in the local areas by a manager, usually a social worker.
3. Functional monitoring, whereby all operational control is delegated to the local organizers, with the central administration responsible for advising, planning, and overseeing the delivery of services.

The "attachment" and "functional monitoring" models are the most prevalent. In the London area, most local home help organizers both administer the program and assess needs for other services such as meals on wheels and day care. In other regions they have more or less direct service responsibilities, depending upon where they are placed in the local social services departments. When management is concentrated in the central office, the assessment and organization of the daily work tends to rest with the local staff in subdistrict offices.

The central government is only peripherally involved in the actual operation of home help services. In addition to grants, it provides general guidelines, leaving to the local authorities the discretion to develop their own programs. Moreover, the central government collects data only on the quantity and not on the quality of services.

Referrals and Determination of Need for Services

Most referrals for home help come from social agencies or from physicians, although many are also initiated by the individual or the family. Upon referral, the home help organizer or the social service worker assesses the extent of services needed. The organizer usually evaluates the degree of physical disability, mental status, previous standards of personal and household care, and the condition of the household. There are no standardized uniform assessment instruments, a fact that often leads to inevitable discrepancies over the need or right for services.

There are basically two types of home help cases: short- and long-term. Short-term cases are reviewed at the end of a designated time limit, while long-term cases have no planned reviews or reassessments. Once services have been initiated, reassessments are rare and are made only if a new problem surfaces or if the client requests it.

Funding for Home Help

Local (municipal or county) authorities decide the level of funding they will allocate for social services, including the home help program. In some areas home help is free, while in others it is free only to recipients of supplementary income benefits. When charges are made, they are based either on a flat weekly rate or on a fee per visit. However, it is debatable as to whether it is cost-effective to charge fees at all. Charges are based on a means test of income, and approximately 70 percent of the elderly fall below the means, which entitles them to free services. The expense of assessing and collecting revenues on the remaining 30 percent may well outweigh the amount collected.

A government study on the cost-effectiveness of twenty-five community care programs (Audit Commission for Local Authorities, 1986) found that estimates of costs were inaccurate as they did not include or measure all of the resources involved in the provision of care. Furthermore, adequate community care often depends on the availability of families, friends, and neighbors, whose investments in time and services are difficult to cost out. With higher rates of dependency, particularly among persons living alone and in need of many services, community care may not necessarily be as cost-effective as residential care.

The net cost of a home help hour varies greatly throughout the country. A study conducted by the Social Services Inspectorate (Department of Health and Social Security, 1987) on a sample of eight departments throughout the country found costs ranging from £2.10 to £3.30 an hour, with an average cost of £2.70 ($4.86). Overall, the eight authorities spent 30 million pounds on home care services in 1984–85, which accounted for 12.4 percent of their total social services budgets. Between 1980 and 1985, their home help expenditures increased by 21 percent, compared to only a 13 percent increase in all other social services during the same period. Nationally, social service expenditures on home help range from 13 to almost 40 percent of all expenditures on the elderly (Department of Health and Social Security, 1987). Furthermore, the provision of home helps ranges from less than seven to forty-four full-time home help workers for every one thousand persons over the age of seventy-five. These differences reflect the diversity of local policies and program emphases in community care.

A comparison of the cost of community home care to other types of care is shown in the following table:

Typical Costs in 1986 Prices (in Pounds) by Care Setting for an Older Person

	Pounds per Week	(U.S.$)
Community Care—Home Care	97.35	$175.23
Residential Care		
A) Local Authority	133.25	239.85
B) Private	138.55	249.39
Hospital	294.75	530.55

Source: Department of Health and Social Security, 1987

District Nurses

District nurses or home nurses provide skilled nursing care to persons in the community. They are usually attached to a general practitioner or a group of practitioners and work as a part of a district nursing team. The role of the nurse includes assessing the needs of patients and their families, supervising other health providers, monitoring the quality of care, and, often, arranging for other support services.

Requests for a district nurse's visit can be made by a general practitioner, social service worker, home help organizer, or the family itself. Approximately 20 percent of the elderly are visited by a district nurse during the year. Moreover, persons over seventy-five years of age receive more than three times as many services from district nurses as those between sixty-five and seventy-four years. The services usually include injections, changing dressings, and health checks (Office of Population Censuses and Surveys, 1982).

Because the nurses are primarily involved in medical care and the home helps provide a broader spectrum of services, coordination between the two programs does not appear to be a problem. Moreover, as the nurses tend to be overworked with large caseloads, there is little resistance to having the home help organizers manage the individual case.

Family and Home Care

Government policies recognize the role of the family in community care through two major benefits. The attendance allowance is payable to persons who are being cared for at home and who require assistance due to mental or physical disability. Persons needing care both day and night received £30.95 a week in 1987, while those requiring only day care were allocated £20.65 per week. Sixty percent of the beneficiaries are over the age of sixty-five, with 41 percent of them claiming the higher allowance rate (Department of Health and Social Security, 1987).

An invalid-care allowance is payable to persons who are under pensionable age, provided they look after a disabled person. The beneficiary must be looking after someone who qualifies for the attendance allowance and must spend a minimum of thirty-five hours every week caring for that person. The weekly rate of the allowance in 1987 was £23.25, plus an extra £13.90 for the dependent adult. In 1986–87 10,500 persons received this allowance. Families are not required to contribute to the costs of home help care, but they are encouraged to continue assisting the frail older relative.

Hospital and Community Care

Many hospitals have established liaison nurses to coordinate the admission and discharge of elderly patients. Their specific roles include exchanging information with community agencies concerning resources that will be needed at discharge. Unfortunately, such liaisons have not been initiated in all areas of the country, and as a consequence many patients are kept in the hospital unnecessarily until home care can be secured. There is also a risk is that they may be released without adequate provision for their needs.

Coordination of Services

There are more than two-hundred health authorities in the country funded by the national Department of Health and Social Security. In many areas the health districts under these authorities overlap with several social service departments that receive separate funding. Furthermore, each social service department and health district designs its own plans for services, which may or may not complement the others (Zwick, 1985).

Efforts to coordinate health and social services have been made through the financing of joint consultation committees and joint finance projects. Under Section 10 of the National Health Services Reorganization Act of 1973, health and local authorities, responsible for social services, were required to coordinate their programs.

In 1974 joint consultative committees were established to advise these local planning and coordinating groups. To further assist with their joint planning, a unified method of financing was also instituted. It was primarily designed to support specific social service demonstrations that would also benefit the local health service as a form of "total care." Joint financing is also available for a limited time to initiate a new project, but local authorities must prove that the project will be continued at the end of the finance period with funding from local revenues. Because of this requirement, joint planning has not been as successful as initially envisioned.

Overall, the coordination of services between the home helps and the other health and social services depends upon the individual departments, their interests, and their abilities to work together. The recurring problem is that many elderly persons require both nursing and social services, but not all authorities have policies and practices for providing these coordinated services (Department of Health and Social Security, 1987).

THE NETHERLANDS

Types of Service

Two nongovernmental organizations, the Central Home Help Association and the National Cross Association responsible for home nursing, are the national "umbrella" providers of home care services. The first of these was established under voluntary religious auspices, with the intent to assist families in which the mother was temporarily incapacitated. Since the 1970s, its emphasis has changed, and today more than half its clients are older persons (Central Council of Home Helps, 1985).

Home help provides domestic and personal support to any person who, due to illness, convalescence, frailty, disability, psychosocial or interpersonal problems, is unable to perform household tasks or requires personal care. Home help workers assist with cleaning, laundry, meal preparation, and shopping as well as personal care, such as bathing and dressing. In certain parts of the country, such as Amsterdam, the home helps are also permitted to administer medications and give routine injections. The home helps may also provide counseling and health education. Basically, the same services are offered throughout the country, although in some areas, care may be extended to twenty-four hours a day, seven days a week.

Organization of the Home Help System

There are presently 250 local home help associations in Holland, most of which are organized into private, nonprofit agencies. Each organization has an autonomous administrative board that sets its own operating policy. These organizations are federated under a national umbrella unit, the already-mentioned Central Home Help Association, which gives technical assistance and lobbies for its consultants in the legislature.

The central government has instituted a home-help services grant scheme, which provides guidelines regarding the basic administrative structure for the services and the conditions for receiving funds. Each organization receives a governmental allocation based on a population formula. The associations also charge fees for their services based on a sliding scale; persons who cannot afford to pay can apply to the government for additional assistance. The government's intervention in the services is limited to a biannual auditing of the home help records. Apart from this, there is no interference in the local operation of the programs, although associations must allocate 75 percent of their funds to direct services.

Coverage

Home help services are used by 12 percent of the elderly population, but this age group constitutes 64 percent of the national caseload of the home help service (Kastelein and Schouten, 1986). There are regional variations in the use of home helps. It is estimated that in Amsterdam, as many as 40 percent of the population over sixty-five years of age receive home help services. Many of these persons would be in institutions if the home helps were not available, because of the lack of familial support. The need for the service lessens in eastern and southern Holland, where there are larger and closer family networks with more informal assistance.

Because of the high demand for services in Amsterdam and other large cities, waiting lists of 60 to 150 persons per district are common. The probiem is compounded by the low wages for the home help workers. In urban areas characterized by high employment rates, the salaries of the agencies are not competitive with those of other industries. This problem tends to lessen in the rural areas.

There is no standardized or definitive point at which a physician, nurse, or home care organizer recommends institutional care rather than home help. In some areas the recommendation for institutionalization is made when the medical problems are too great or costly, while in other areas that have developed home hospice care, the extent of required care is not a precipitating or deciding factor. The recent addition of weekend and night care and the removal of the previous limit of forty hours a week of service have made it possible for many very ill elderly who previously would have been institutionalized to continue being cared for at home.

Models of Home Help Care

Local associations may select their own organizational model of home help, provided that the administrative overhead does not exceed 25 percent of the budget. The standard prototype model consists of the division of geographic domain into smaller districts. Each of the latter is assigned a manager, who oversees one or several team leaders and one or several teams of home helps.

Amsterdam is divided into twelve such districts, each headed by a district manager who leads two to three teams. In comparison, Leiden, a small city near Amsterdam, consists of only three districts and three teams. Each district in Leiden has nine part-time leaders who supervise two hundred home help workers each. In addition to the team leaders, there is a coordinator for each district who meets with the nine leaders daily to allocate the schedule of cases for the day. The intention is to simplify this system by having ten workers assigned to twenty to thirty clients, and then letting these workers make their own service plans. The simplified scheme would give more responsibility to the individual worker in charge of the case. The role of the leaders could be reduced, because they would meet with the workers weekly rather than daily, while the workers would meet more frequently in teams. In addition, the team concept would enable the workers to substitute more easily for each other.

Determination of Need for Services

Persons can be referred to home help by any source, including themselves. The request is evaluated by the district leader or manager, who decides what services are needed. The assessment is made on a standardized form developed by the Central Home Help Association and used throughout the country. The form assesses the physical and mental functions of the client as well as the availability for informal supports who might contribute some assistance. The aim is to provide only assistance that is not available from any other source. When there is a waiting list for assistance, priority is given to those who could not remain in their homes without immediate help.

The leader determines the number of hours to be allotted to each case. The average number of hours of service an older person receives is between four and five hours per week. The program attempts to be flexible and to meet individual needs. As a result, home help workers may make several visits to a single client in the same day. Care may also be provided at night, with visits being made at late as 11 P.M. In short-term situations, such as in terminal care or in an acute illness, twenty-four-hour care may also be offered.

Clients are normally reassessed every six months. However, reviews may occur more frequently at the manager's discretion or when a worker recommends that a reassessment be made.

Coordination of Services

It is not uncommon for elderly persons to be visited by both a home help and a Cross Association nurse. It is obvious, then, that the personal tasks that these care givers perform, such as bathing and the administration of medications, may overlap. There are no uniform criteria for deciding which worker or agency takes primary responsibility for a client or who will perform specific tasks. The decision is made on a case-by-case basis by the district managers of each program. As may be expected, this lack of coordination often creates administrative difficulties in the provision of services.

If the patient's problems are primarily medical, the case will probably be supervised by the home nurse. On the other hand, if the home help was working with the client prior to the nurse's involvement, the home help may continue overseeing the case.

Despite the lack of formal linkage between the programs, informal strategies have been developed to prevent disruption or tension among services. In some areas the managers of the local home help service and the Cross Association meet weekly or monthly to discuss common cases. These meetings may also include the individual home helps and nurses assigned to specific clients. Agencies that have frequent informal inter-actions such as these are better prepared to deal with problems as they emerge. In order to further enhance program coordination, the home helps and the nurses usually keep a logbook in the client's home in which they each record the tasks they have completed and any problems that may have been observed.

Unfortunately, efforts to coordinate agencies are not uniform through-out the country. In order to rectify the situation, the Cross Association and the Central Home Help Association are planning to merge. The goal is to create a single agency, which will increase both programs' effec-tiveness and reduce the overlap and duplication of services.

Coordination with Hospitals

Home help agencies are closely connected with the hospitals. If a hos-pitalized elderly person will be requiring home help care at discharge, a hospital social worker telephones the district leader prior to the patient's leaving the hospital. At this time, the leader visits the home to conduct an environmental assessment and may also interview the patient in the hospital if help will be needed immediately.

If the patient had home help prior to hospital admission, the home help worker usually contacts the hospital social worker. In most instances, the same home help will care for the patient at discharge.

Amsterdam has initiated a "flying brigade" of home helps who provide care immediately upon discharge on an emergency basis. This team covers the entire city and is intended to counteract the problems that can occur when anticipated discharges are made. To date, this program has proven very effective in reducing discontinuities of services between hospital and home.

The National Cross Association

The National Cross Association, a national community nursing agency, is the second major program in home care. The Dutch Cross Association was founded in 1875, initially to deal with contagious diseases. In sub-sequent years, local associations sponsored by various churches were established throughout the country to assist persons needing public health nursing. These associations continued to work independently at the local level until 1938, when the Federation of Protestant Christian Associations of District Nursing was established. In 1974, these organizations merged into the National Cross Work Center, and in 1977 this became the Na-tional Cross Association.

Presently, the National Cross Association is a federation of fifteen provincial Cross Associations with approximately two hundred local agencies. The total number of employees is over 16,000, of which over one-third are district nurses. The national association receives contracts from the central government, establishes service-related policies, lobbies with the government, and provides technical assistance to the provincial associations (National Cross Association, 1988).

The central government defines the services that the Cross Association must perform under its contracts. Within this broad framework, local variations and innovations are permitted if funds are available. The government collects data on expenditures and services. Individual agencies are invited to make recommendations to the government regarding their unique needs and problems, although there is no guarantee that these needs will be met.

In principle, the same services are offered throughout the country. A majority of associations provide twenty-four-hour service and evening visits to meet needs of the chronically or terminally ill. The present dilemma faced by the organization is whether to give greater priority to preventive rather than curative care. Whereas some local associations allocate 20 percent of their services to preventive care, others limit it to only 10 percent. Budget restrictions and growing community needs make it difficult to provide both kinds of care. The decision about these priorities rests with the local managers.

Organizational Structure

The National Cross Association divides the nation's provinces into districts, which are further divided into basic units. Each unit covers the care of a population ranging between sixteen thousand and sixty thousand persons, and is headed by a district nurse who supervises a team of qualified district nurses and nurse's aides. The provincial organization is responsible for the overall administration and support of these units.

Coverage and Funding

It is estimated that 15.8 percent of the elderly living alone in the community have had contact at one time or another with a district nurse (Kastelein and Schouten, 1986). The association estimates that 58 percent of the population eighty years of age and older has received care from Cross nurses. Coverage is universal, and everyone requiring care is automatically eligible to receive it.

The Exceptional Medical Expenses Act mandates the central government to pay for 80 percent of the association's service-related costs. Although the need for nursing care has continued to escalate, the association has received only small budgetary increments of 1 to 2 percent per year. As with the home help services, this reveals further ambivalence and inconsistency in the government's commitment to a policy of domiciliary care.

Persons receiving nursing care pay a small annual fee to the association of 40.50 guilders ($19.00) per year. This entitles them to all of the care they may require without limitations on the length of service. In practice, however, three hours of nursing care per day is generally the daily maximum.

Coordination with Hospital Care

The Cross nurses, as primary providers of nursing care in the community, are expected to coordinate their work with the nursing staff in the hospitals. However, this relationship is not equally successful throughout the country. Ward nurses in hospitals are responsible for the discharge planning and for contacting the district Cross nurse if a patient will require further assistance at home. The Cross nurse may then go to the hospital to discuss the discharge plans and to make a further assessment of the patient's needs.

The association has developed a system with two hospitals in Amsterdam in which Cross patients have "procedure" cards that they take with them to the hospital to notify the staff about their affiliation with the agency. This has improved communication between the Cross nurses and the discharge planners and is being extended to more hospitals, making it possible for nurses to get to the home of a discharged patient immediately, if so needed. In some locations the Cross district nurse carries a beeper so that the hospital can inform her if a patient requiring urgent care has been discharged.

MANITOBA, CANADA

Scope and Limits of Home Care Services

The province of Manitoba offers a wide array of health and social services under the rubric of home care. This includes multidisciplinary assessments, nursing visits, homemaking, home maintenance, personal care, respite care, oxygen therapy, meals, intravenous or hyperalimentation therapy, enterostomal therapy, and day care.

To limit costs, services are provided at the most essential level, and total expenditures may not exceed the costs of equivalent care levels in an institution, except under special circumstances. When there are questions regarding the eligibility of a specific client, the regional care coordinator makes the final decision.

In all other instances, the individual case coordinator decides which services should be offered.

Home Care and Nursing Homes

The Continuing Care Program continues a sequence of long-term care services with home care as the entry point, which for some persons may eventually lead to the nursing home. The same standardized assessment instrument is used for both modes of care—home care and nursing home—with home care as the option usually preferred. Since both systems are funded by the government, there is no competition for clients. Moreover, the lengthy waiting lists for nursing home beds, have fostered this sector's interest in keeping patients in the community.

Patients can enter nursing homes only after an assessment panel composed of the regional program coordinator, senior nurse or social worker, physician, and often a representative of the nursing home has determined that they require institutional care. The key factor in the panel's decision is often the informal supports available, since many persons requiring extensive care can still be managed in the community. This sociological reality has altered the definition of "risk of institutionalization" and made it contingent on the available supports rather than on the patient's degree of functional incapacity.

If the panel decides that the person can stay in the community without undue risk, he or she will not be approved for a nursing home even if this conflicts with the family's or the patient's desires. The panel will also consider the point at which the family may be unable to provide adequate care. Accurate social assessments are thus essential to the operation of both the home care and the nursing home programs.

Entering the System—Referrals and Assessment

Referrals for home care can be made to the regional offices by any person or source. A standardized assessment instrument is used throughout the province to examine the applicant's medical, social, and psychological status, cognitive functioning, and the informal social supports available. It identifies the household, health, personal, and social assistance required for the individual to remain at home, distinguishing those tasks that the family can perform from those for which formal assistance is required. In most instances, the assessment is done in the individual's home, although it may also take place in the hospital. Family members are usually included or consulted during the assessment process.

If the assessment is made by a team of a nurse and a social worker, one of these professionals, depending on the dominant needs of the client, will become the case coordinator. This person decides, among other things, the number of hours of care to be provided. The home care services are defined as supplemental because they provide only what the client, family, or other informal supports cannot offer. Thus patients receiving home care immediately after leaving the hospital are reassessed a few weeks after their discharge. In general, these reassessments take place every three months or less, depending on the effectiveness or results of the home care plan. The patient's physician may also be contacted at the time of the reassessment.

The Care Plan

Individualized care plans are based on the preceding diagnostic assessment. They include both the services needed in the home and those that can be obtained from existing community programs. Moreover, the plan identifies services that can be purchased from other agencies, services, or contractors. It may also suggest alterations or adaptations in the house that will enable the individual to function independently for a longer period of time. The plan outlines both the goals that are to be achieved through the intervention and the schedule of reassessments.

Coordination

Coordination does not constitute a problem in the Manitoba system, since all services derive from or through a single agency. In fact, coordination is built into the entire system, from the central office through the direct provision of services in the regional and local offices.

Although the Continuing Care Program is centrally administered, the delivery of services is decentralized. The rationale underlying this format is that (1) fragmentation of services is wasteful, inefficient, and inimical to the welfare of the most vulnerable; (2) health, welfare, and social factors are interdependent; and (3) decentralized assessment and delivery are best able to respond to local conditions and needs (Berdes, 1987). Thus within the guidelines of the Continuing Care Program, regional offices have some latitude in the design and implementation of their programs.

The regional continuing-care coordinators monitor and review all cases in their respective jurisdictions and also collect information, prepare budgets, and plan programs. They also monitor the performance of the 120 case coordinators responsible for direct services outside of Winnipeg. Within Winnipeg, there are three coordinating regional agencies, two of which deal with long-term care (sixty days or more) and one, the Victorian Order of Nurses, that covers short-term care upon discharge from a hospital.

Case coordinators procure the services needed by their clients. They consequently organize and manage the direct services, including homemaking, personal care, day care, respite, physical therapy, occupational therapy, social work, and nursing. Physical and occupational therapy are not part of the Continuing Care Program battery of services, but may be purchased from nonprofit agencies.

Home Care and Hospital Care

The home care offices staffed by the Victorian Order of Nurses (V.O.N.) initiate the care plans for the first two weeks following hospital discharges. V.O.N. coordinates the case in question for a period of up to three months. At this point, a coordinator from the Continuing Care Program rather than a supervisor from the Victorian Order of Nurses monitors the patient. If in fact it appears that long-term care is needed after discharge, the referral is made directly to the Continuing Care Program in Winnipeg.

The short-term V.O.N. home care program is available on a twenty-four-hour basis seven days a week. There is no limit in fact, to the number of visits, and patients are not required to cover any of the costs of care. Visits average around $25.00 (Canadian) each. Long-term patients are reassessed every three months, and short-term cases are reviewed every four to five weeks.

Each Winnipeg hospital has a home care office staffed by V.O.N. nurses. These nurses attend regular hospital rounds on the wards in order to elicit referrals. The goal is to begin planning for discharge at the time of admission and to ensure that services will be immediately available, without waiting lists.

In the short-term home care (V.O.N.) program, four nursing supervisors monitor twenty-five to thirty home care nurses through daily meetings. Close supervision is essential to assure program effectiveness. Standards for nursing care are based upon a manual of procedures. Physicians maintain an important role in the service as they may refer to the home care program and are expected to review patient medications every three months. The physicians are notified immediately if any changes are observed in the patient.

All of the V.O.N. home care nurses are registered nurses who receive salaries comparable to those in hospitals. As of June 1988 there were approximately 108 full-time and 30 part-time nurses. Together they average eight to nine visits per day and are able to meet the needs of the population. The working conditions are relatively better than for nurses working in institutions, a fact which makes community care more attractive.

The Continuing Care Program has a unique link with the Victorian Order of Nurses. Although the program has no direct supervisory power over V.O.N., it does purchase their services, and as such V.O.N. must adhere to existing program mandates, criteria, and guidelines. Each nursing visit, as well as the salaries of the discharge planners, is covered by the Continuing Care Program. This cooperation, whereby the fiscal agency has funding and program authority over its direct service counterpart, produces results because both programs respond to similar mandates and policy guidelines. However, the V.O.N. primarily assesses the patient's medical needs, consistent with its short-term, posthospital discharge philosophy, while the Continuing Care Program makes a broader evaluation of the patient's social and psychological condition. It may, therefore, accept a case which had not met the V.O.N.'s more restrictive criteria.

The relationship between the V.O.N. and the Continuing Care Program may be further complicated by the increasingly sophisticated care required by many patients. As care becomes more expensive, the question arises whether other private firms will be hired to provide it or whether it will remain the sole domain of the Victorian Order of Nurses.

An advantage of the relationship between the V.O.N. and the Continuing Care Program is that it fully integrates home care with the hospital. This allows discharge planning to be fully comprehensive and part of the original treatment plan.

Urban-area hospitals outside Winnipeg have designated care coordinators who serve as liaisons with their local area Continuing Care office. In rural areas, if there is no hospital coordinator the hospital nurse contacts the local care coordinator regarding each patient's discharge needs. The care coordinator, in fact, may visit the hospital weekly to assess patients and determine who will be requiring home care.

Hospitals thus ensure that discharge plans are in place and will keep patients until adequate discharge plans are instituted and implemented. Ideally, discharge planning is initiated at the time of admission. However, even though services may be provided seven days a week, the care coordinator, or the required resources, is not always immediately available. These facts also contribute to lengthening a patient's hospital stay.

Presently, the case coordinators in Winnipeg South average 130 cases each, exceeding both the optimal caseload size of 90 cases and the provincial program standard for staffing. These large caseloads make it difficult to conduct in-depth assessments and effective family problem-solving interventions.

The case coordinators visit their clients every two to three months to monitor all aspects of the care plan. They make referrals to other agencies, keep track of their clients in day hospitals, and oversee the entire service package. If a client requires nursing care, the coordinator either purchases the service from the Victorian Order of Nurses or requests a

licensed practical nurse. The case coordinator also assesses clients for
nursing home placement and presents these cases to the panel in charge
of such determinations of eligibility for institutional care.

Winnipeg offers a home orderly service for cases that require frequent
services of short duration, that is, fifteen minutes per visit. These or-
derlies assist with personal care and provide many of the same functions
as the home attendants, but for shorter time periods, usually less than
an hour per day. The tasks performed include assisting persons to transfer
from bed to wheelchair, to bathe, and to dress. It is an important service
because it frees home attendants to provide more extensive care in the
client's home.

Continuing Care Program—Winnipeg South

It may be useful to examine the structure and organization of one of
the largest regions in order to review the Continuing Care Program. In
Winnipeg the program is divided into three administrative regions. Each
region has a regional continuing care coordinator who directs several
teams of case coordinators for assessment and services coordination. In
addition, there are resource coordinators, who recruit and supervise the
direct service staff.

The Winnipeg South region has four teams of case coordinators in each
of its two office locations. Each consists of a nurse (B. N.) and a social
worker (B.S.W.). The team assesses each patient's needs and then obtains
or provides all of their required services. As discussed earlier, all home
care services—social work, personal care, nursing, therapy (occupational
and physical), and home help—are either provided directly or purchased
through the Office of Continuing Care. However, the home help and
personal care services are coordinated and monitored by the resource
coordinators in each of the district offices.

If the assessment indicates the need for home help services, the case
coordinator sends an assignment sheet and service authorization form to
the resource coordinator, who then assigns the home support workers.
As these support workers notice changes in a client, they must report
them to their supervisor, the resource coordinator, who in turn reports
them to the case coordinator.

ARGENTINA

Home Care and Health Care

Originally inspired by the British model of comprehensive health care
but also incorporating some locally distinctive features, the Comprehen-

sive Medical Care Program (PAMI) for the aged was organized by the federal government in three levels.

The first, or primary, level consists of direct physician's and dentist's services available to residents of each of the geographically designated districts. The entire country is divided into twenty-nine major administrative regions, or PAMI's "delegations." Each is in turn subdivided in districts or catchment areas, designed for easy access to services. The program is federally operated and financed, with no participation of the provincial governments, city authorities, or the voluntary sector in its oversight, design, funding, or actual implementation. An incipient trend towards sporadic and complementary home care services, however, has been slowly evolving outside the federal domain in recent years, for the most part under municipal auspices. Each elderly resident can select a primary physician and dentist, but only from a list of PAMI-contracted health professionals in his or her district of residence.

The capital city of Buenos Aires, with a population of over 8 million people and over 1.5 million elderly, is a self-contained PAMI delegation, divided into ten districts. The original intent was that each district serve, on the average, an eligible population of 100,000 to 150,000 elderly.

Each district's headquarters provides outpatient medical services, psychiatry, dentistry, nursing care, laboratory tests, and diagnostic evaluations. The latter are needed to authorize inpatient and institutional services as well as home care services.

Home care is provided by home nurses and "domiciliary auxiliaries" (home attendants). Both categories of workers are employed full-time by PAMI's district offices. They draw full fringe benefits and, in an economy characterized by endemic underemployment, they also enjoy a substantial measure of job security and stability.

The pivotal component of the health care system for the aged is the already mentioned primary physician (*médico de cabecera*) selected by the elderly beneficiaries from a list of professionals in their districts. These are not, however, PAMI's regular employees, but private practitioners contracted to take on a caseload that may range between five hundred and one thousand potential users. They are compensated on a capitation basis for the total caseload, regardless of the volume of actual utilization of their services. Each operates, consequently, as a mini–Health Maintenance Organization (HMO). At the time of the study, in August 1988, they received a monthly fee of six *australes* per participant, equivalent then to $0.60. There are no prescribed limits as to the times an older person may see his or her primary physician. The visits take place in the doctor's private offices, but the patient is also entitled to receive home visits in cases of severe infirmity or physical incapacitation. The primary physicians, therefore, initiate the home treatment process, which later on they may delegate to home care nurses and the home attendants.

The second level of health care consists of short-stay hospital care for acute conditions. It includes specialized medical and dental consultation, diagnosis and treatment, surgery, emergency treatment, and nursing and homemaker services after discharge. Hospitals are reimbursed by the National Institute of Social Services for Retirees and Pensioners on the basis of a uniform fees schedule, periodically adjusted for inflation, and substantially similar to the prospective-payment system prevalent in the United States under Medicare's DRG provisions.

The third level comprises nursing home care for prolonged or indefinite geriatric or psychogeriatric institutionalization. Similarly to the first and second levels, it rests on contractual arrangements with privately owned facilities to whom the National Institute will pay a monthly subsidy or fixed assignment per eligible patient, actually an established ceiling of benefits. The patient and/or the family are responsible for covering the difference between the actual billings and the established reimbursement rate. There is no requirement that patients "spend down" their assets, but they must apply part of their social security benefits to pay for the nursing home costs.

PAMI's comprehensive services include 100 percent coverage for inpatient care medications and 50 to 70 percent for outpatient pharmaceuticals. Anticancer and imported drugs are distributed free of charge, as are pacemakers and prosthesis items. PAMI is also engaged in the provision of protective shelter, congregate housing, home improvement services, health education, day care, and leisure and recreation centers. Rarely are so many programs subsumed under a single agency. The unmistakable intent was to coordinate all health and social services, while leaving the income maintenance programs in a separate institute also within the State Ministry of Social Action.

Home care may also be initiated at the so-called secondary or hospitalization level, particularly after discharge. Nursing home care—the tertiary level—is hard to get because there simply are not enough beds available. It tends to be unaffordable for those who cannot pay the difference between the nursing home charges and the rate authorized by the National Institute. Home care services become, then, the most likely alternative at this tertiary level.

Home care may be initiated at any of the three levels of health care, but it is the primary care physician who usually initiates the request for home care services. This request is submitted to a PAMI district office, where it is reviewed by both the nursing and the social work supervisors. In the eventuality of emerging or new medical problems, the case is referred to an assessment team that includes, at least in principle, the primary physician. Decisions are not made immediately, and with the growing demand for services, it may take up to fifteen days before the district will issue an authorization for home care. The district nurse supervisor draws the service plan. For each patient, services may require both nursing and homemaking personnel. These home care services are provided only during the day and evening hours, from 7 A.M. to 8 P.M., but do not include weekend days. In the eventuality of an emergency during the night or on weekends, the district office dispatches ambulances or a physician. Once again, the home care response may involve physician participation in the field itself, but only in the case of a major crisis warranting what is considered an exceptional measure.

For the second level of care, that is, hospitalization, each of PAMI's district offices has instituted a coordinating center to follow up on discharged patients. It is basically a case management function, but it is limited to medical and social work service inputs. The actual discharge is decided jointly by the hospital's physician responsible for the case and his or her counterpart at the coordinating center. Based upon their assessment, the district office may set in motion a special round of home care services.

The Role of the Primary Physician

The Argentine model is the most medically oriented of all those under scrutiny in this study. In contrast with the Norwegian approach, for instance, which legitimizes any source of referral for home care including the patients themselves, the physician in Argentina acts as the exclusive gatekeeper. Moreover, the gatekeeper is not just any physician but only the primary one contracted by the National Institute. The initial policy blueprint called for the following operational procedures:

1. The primary physician authorizes the provision of home care and leads the home care team by conducting home visits when the patient's condition so warrants it.
2. Similarly, the primary physician makes diagnostic home rounds.
3. The primary physician provides continuity of service by coordinating with other services. This is reminiscent of the American case management model.

In addition, the policy incorporates the idea of "home hospitalization," that is, the systematic continuation of services following hospital discharge. It calls for the secondary physician, namely, the hospital practitioner responsible for the case, the primary—or general—practitioner, and the specialists at the district office to design, set in motion, and follow up a treatment plan in the patient's own home, following the hospital treatment.

The day-to-day experience, however, does not conform to the rather ambitious expectations of the home hospitalization model. To begin with, the primary physicians are sorely underpaid, and in an economy of endemic inflation, a three- to four-week delay in reimbursement could well signify a 25 to 30 percent loss in the purchase power of the outstanding bills. The country's economic woes thus weigh heavily on the medical practitioners and inevitably contribute to their demoralization. Primary physicians react to these crushing economic disadvantages by curbing their services. They begin by cutting or refusing altogether to make home visits. They often invoke the justifiable fear of muggings and assaults in high-crime areas as the reason for that refusal. They insist that the Institute should authorize home visits by emergency doctors only, traveling in an ambulance. It goes without saying that a private practitioner who carries a caseload of nearly one thousand registered patients as a second job can hardly provide continuity of care, even to the fraction of patients in active treatment.

A View from a District

While aggregate statistics of service utilization for the entire program covering the twenty-nine national delegations are unattainable, an in-depth examination of records for a single district (District 4) in the Buenos Aires delegation revealed that it included fifty-two thousand registered elderly participants, and that they were assigned to ninety primary physicians. The total number of units of service performed in 1987 by these district primary physicians was 200,566. This represented a yearly average of almost 4 units per eligible older person. Conversely, each primary physician performed 2,228 units of service, or an average of 185 a month. Home visits were tabulated separately, adding only 8,270 units of service for the entire year, or an annual average of 91 per physician, in effect less than 2 per week. It may be observed, therefore, that only 2.2 percent of all units of service took place as medical home visits.

Nonmedical home care visits totaled 13,605 for the same year. It is also important to observe that they fall in three categories: the already mentioned home nursing and domiciliary auxiliary services (homemaking) plus physical therapy, a separate service that emphasizes rehabilitation treatment. It was rather surprising to notice that the latter is the leading category, with almost 6,000 units of service, followed by an almost equal number—5,750—of home nursing services, leaving a rather miniscule proportion, only 1,900 units, for homemaking services. The reality is that most homemaking is still performed by relatives. All home visits, both medical and nonmedical, total 21,875 in one year. Nearly 38 percent were physician visits; 27 percent were visits by physical therapists; practical nurses conducting home nursing visits came in third place with 26 percent; and homemakers came a distant last, with 9 percent of the total.

The total number of actual beneficiaries of home nursing was 686 for the entire year, and 396 of them remained as active cases by the end of 1987. Those receiving homemaker services numbered 429 patients, with 356 listed in the active rolls at the end of the year. In manpower terms, there were six home nurses for the district. They were practical nurses, or nurse's auxiliaries, as they are called in Argentina. Homemakers declined in number from six full-time equivalencies to barely three at the end of the year. This reduction was due to retirements, but vacancies were not filled due to stringent cost-containment policies. It may be also observed that the number of nursing units of service provided at the district's office surpassed those delivered at home. They totaled 6,245 and benefited 992 registered elderly.

There are some obvious conclusions that may be derived from the statistics on District 4. To begin with, the emphasis in home care services is tilted in the direction of physicians' visits, followed by the less traditional but highly professionalized physical therapy. Even if homemaker and home nursing services are entirely free, their utilization is rather limited simply because primary physicians—the gatekeepers who prescribe home care services—seemingly give low priority to these ancillary services. Also, patients may be discouraged, given the presumed long and uncertain waiting periods until the services are authorized. Because of the district office's rather accessible location, many patients choose to go there to obtain outpatient nursing services—nebulizations, injections, heart pressure monitoring, changes of dressings, and so forth—rather than wait for such services at home. This is the way PAMI prefers it anyway, for obvious cost-reduction reasons.

CONCLUSION

In all six countries home care services include domestic help, personal care, nursing, and medical care. In general, home help and home nursing are the two dominant types of home services available to the elderly. Moreover, home help may even be further divided into regular domestic assistance and heavy-duty cleaning. Home care services may thus include dressing and personal care, assistance with medications, shopping, cleaning, laundry, meal preparation, errands, socialization, and escorting.

There is a varying emphasis on health status as the main requirement for eligibility. In most countries, social deprivation may also justify access to home care. The programmatic distinction between home help and home nursing is giving way in some countries to the experimentation with a more syncretic model, whereby home helps are trained to take on some nursing aide services and work in teams with nursing personnel. Professional boundaries thus give way to a more undifferentiated or generic form of home assistance.

Coordination with hospitals may be initiated at the very moment of admission or close to discharge. In some instances the hospital head nurse contacts the district homemaker or home nurse supervisor to facilitate continuity of care. A second model consists of a special liaison nurse employed to coordinate the discharge. A third variation entails a multidisciplinary team within the hospital, also incorporating the patient's primary-care physician. This team designs a new plan of care to be initiated at discharge.

Assessments and care plans are usually made by either a nurse or home help supervisor who is often a social worker. In many programs, the person making the assessment becomes the client's case manager. This manager may be the first person to receive the referral. When there are no clear criteria for deciding whether a home help or nurse should officiate as the case manager, there is the potential for conflict between the two occupational groups. Some countries seek to resolve or neutralize the impending conflict by allocating primary case responsibility to one or the other occupation.

5

Manpower

The effectiveness of home care programs is directly associated with the quality and competence of the personnel providing the services. All the countries studied share with the United States problems in recruiting and retaining qualified home care workers. This chapter examines the roles and duties assigned to these workers, their training, and the strategies put into effect to ensure the stability and continuity of this specialized workforce.

NORWAY

Home care has been historically shaped in Norway by a nursing-medical model. Most of the country's 46,000 professional nurses are hospital employees. In 1986, 4,142, or less than 10 percent of the nurses, worked for county governments, and 56.2 percent of them were in the home care service sector. With decentralization came the move to attend to all patients' needs, and consequently a social dimension has been added. The resulting social model implies that (1) services address the total person, not just the illness; and (2) patients participate in decisions concerning their treatment.

In order to care for the total needs of elderly patients, counties must recruit an adequate number of trained home care workers. Shortages of personnel are serious in the cities, even though there is still an ample supply of paraprofessionals in the rural areas. Some cities and localities have a large immigrant population from countries such as Turkey, Morocco, and Bangladesh. Many immigrant women are being incorporated into the service professions, but this has become a politically sensitive issue, tied to prevailing immigration policies. In other cities, authorities are trying to recruit middle-aged housewives, male workers displaced from technologically obsolete occupations, and students. Thus there is an apparent contradiction between the aspiration of upgrading the image and appeal of home care through professionalization and resorting to manpower sources for whom home care may constitute a last resort and a transient form of employment.

The difficulty of recruiting and retaining home care workers is due to many reasons: the job is physically exhausting, the salaries are low, and there are few opportunities for advancement. Moreover, workers must shoulder too much of an emotional burden, and they lack sufficient training to cope with the new situations. Finally, they work under conditions of relative isolation.

Nurses are more inclined to take on supervisory and administrative positions. The inevitable trend, therefore, is to assign more of the routine tasks such as bathing, dressing simple wounds, and taking blood pressure to the nurse's aides. Physical and occupational therapists are also becoming more integrated in the service, a trend that may facilitate a move away from an emphasis on care to one of prevention and rehabilitation. The home nurse's traditional role is becoming more circumscribed, and some fear that this may jeopardize the quality of care. It may, however, also facilitate the recruitment of more registered nurses, once they perceive that they do not have to carry the entire weight of the service on their shoulders.

District leaders in Oslo are particularly concerned about the recruitment and retention of home helpers. They have laboriously tried to change the perception of home care as a low-status occupation by advocating more liberal benefits. The latter include paid travel time between client and client; a paid half hour for lunch; paid one-and-a-half weekly hours for professional meetings; special allocation of funds for clothing; and leave days, especially for health reasons, for those working more than fifteen weekly hours.

The rate of absenteeism remains consistently high, despite the improvement of benefits. During April of 1988, for instance, districts in Oslo reported a total of 3,059 service hours for the home helpers working 15 to 37 hours a week, counterbalanced by 863 hours of illness, 113 hours of holiday time and 260 hours of personal leave, a total of 1,236 hours. Home helpers working less than 15 hours weekly provided during the same month 3,238 hours of services but reported only 164 hours of illness and no leave time. The total of those working 15 to 37 hours a week was thirty-six. There were in addition seventy-seven part-timers working less than 15 weekly hours.

Elderly clients tend to voice more complaints about workers' absenteeism than about service quality. Conflicts also arise with regard to the task limits imposed on the home helpers. Originally they were not supposed to provide personal care such as bathing, hair washing, cutting toenails or checking on the intake of medicines. These were tasks reserved for the nurse's aides or home health nurses. The role of the home helpers has been gradually expanded in recent years, but it still remains ill defined.

Clients expect workers to wash windows and walls every week, tasks which are explicitly disallowed. Workers complain, in turn, about inappropriate last-minute requests such as food shopping for an entire two-week period when the groceries must be carried by hand to a fourth-floor walk-up apartment. The city administration expects home helpers to exercise more discretion on how to organize their schedules and how to prioritize among competing demands. The district leader assigns new cases to the groups, but each helper is given the authority to decide how long to spend with each client, what specific services to deliver, and who gets priority attention. Home helpers resist this newly won administrative freedom. Many want no part of decision making and the ensuing responsibilities.

Each of Oslo's fourteen city districts must do its own recruiting and cope, in the process, with negative images about home help work. District 2 resorts to relentless outreach publicity: it advertises in the main city dailies, places notices in shops and public places, and targets its announcements to college students who seek part-time, temporary employment. District leaders are confident that the new educational requirements and financial inducements provided to home helpers will bolster their sense of mission and self-esteem. To elevate their status, the city is now requiring that they attend a one-year full-time course, with 60 percent of the time paid at normal wage levels. In return, they must assume the commitment to work for a minimum of one year in home help care.

Regrettably, many fulfill that obligation by switching to the home health care side of home care and become nurse's aides. In this sector there is less physical exertion as well as the prospect of better career advances. Home health nurses used to have authority over home help services. They were subsequently separated and placed on equal footing. However, home health nurses are persistently trying to repossess their position of control. Home help leaders are concerned with the consequent risks of further status demotion. They regard it as not only counter-productive but also paradoxical in a time when public authorities are determined to improve the home helper's image.

Leaders point out that home helpers are the front-liners, who sustain the most intense contact with the client. They provide about 70 percent of all home care services, and their interventions go far beyond concrete services. The moment they step into a client's home, they are confronted with myriad problems: loneliness, depression, alcoholism, dementia, over-medication, and even imminent death. It is not possible in most instances to bring in the specialists necessary to attend to all these needs. Home helpers must resort to their own means of coping. For this reason, home helpers need to receive more systematic training, including instruction in how to communicate orally with individuals and in group conferences, how to do their paperwork, and how to make decisions and back them up properly. The key to their success is more respect, better recognition, and better wages.

The Ministry of Church and Education, in cooperation with the Ministry of Consumer Affairs and Government Administration, has prepared a four-week course (144 hours) for the training of home helps. A correspondence course is also available through the auspices of the Norwegian Correspondence School.

While it is customarily preferred that home helps receive some type of training, this is not mandated by law nor is it a condition of employment. As of 1982, 86 percent had not attended any formal course, only 5.2 percent had completed the four-week course, and 8.6 percent had attended shorter courses.

There are, however, variations across municipalities. Oslo is now requiring that home care supervisors be trained for a full year and be fully compensated during that period.

Norway pioneered in making training available for relatives who assume regular care-giving roles for disabled persons. This is currently available to parents of disabled children, but potentially it may be expanded to also include the relatives of Alzheimer's disease victims. Care givers who leave their regular occupations to care for diseased relatives will be entitled to receive regular compensation as well as retirement pension credits. Some of Norway's experimental long-term care programs have highlighted the need to redefine traditional job categories and articulate novel team approaches to services. Ammerudhjemmet is a case in point.

The Ammerudhjemmet Service Center

Ammerudhjemmet is a comprehensive service center for the aged on the outskirts of Oslo. It was created in 1970 as a religious, nondenominational rehabilitation institute and is, in fact, also designed to train the home helps. Program planners realize the difficulties implicit in this model, but they find that it motivates the home helps by reducing task repetitiveness and promoting professional growth. The initial results indicate a substantial upgrading in skills. Instead of having two workers assigned to each client, that is, a home helper and a home nurse, there is now a single home helper who can also take on many home health functions. The client similarly benefits by relating to a single home care worker.

The administrative staff is clustered in departments assigned to the different geographic districts. Each office is managed by a staff leader, who is not required to be a nurse. This in itself is quite a substantial departure from tradition. Skilled therapists and professionals such as occupational therapists, physical therapists, and social workers are assigned to an interdisciplinary team rather than constituting separate professional departments. They do meet on occasion in distinct professional groups but do not have formal standing as such in the organization.

Ammerudhjemmet espouses the philosophical premise that staying in the home is a person's right and that services must be subordinated to this right. To the cost-effectiveness argument that if people need more than 6.5 hours per week of home care, it would make more economic sense to place them in an institution, the Ammerudhjemmet leaders counter that the very purpose of institutional care needs to be revised. They further claim that nursing home care should be fused and integrated into a comprehensive service model for the area district. Clients could then be brought to the nursing home for a short period of time for rehabilitation by their home helpers and not for permanent institutionalization.

The teams of home help workers assigned to the district eventually rotate and work for a defined period within the nursing home, always as a team. This open-care model is intended to break the dichotomy between community care and nursing home care. Depending on the client's needs, it is sometimes necessary to admit a person for long-term care. The assigned home helper would then work inside the institution until the patient was again discharged. This is defined as a "rubber wall" approach to nursing home care, whereby the institution metaphorically contracts or expands depending on the number of clients admitted. It also increases or decreases the number of staff accordingly.

Staff are drawn from the cadre of district teams. Even with a stable distribution of institutional and community-based clients, those teams are expected to work both inside and out of the institution to signify that they really are invested in the continuum of care. The open-care institution has also adopted an open-door policy whereby it welcomes older persons from the surrounding community to use its facilities as a drop-in center where they can meet friends, dance, have hot meals and search for new pursuits. They also encourage seniors who are community residents to use Ammerudhjemmet's facilities for club and voluntary organizational meetings. Similarly, they provide a meeting place for other independent voluntary organizations serving the aged, and they involve younger persons in intergenerational exchanges.

Ammerudhjemmet operates under contract with the city of Oslo, but it sets its own quality and efficiency standards. It is an experiment in flexibility, because it does not accept the established boundaries between the home help and home nursing professions; nor does it recognize the distinct separation of institutional and home care. The administration accepts part-time home helpers as long as they are motivated and committed. Staff morale is high, as evidenced by a 15 percent turnover rate per year compared to Oslo's 50 percent rate.

Ammerudhjemmet's success hinges on organizational factors such as a better opportunities for upward mobility into team leadership positions, relentless and in-depth training, a greater emphasis on teamwork and support, rotational schedules, and an emphasis on recruitment from its own community. Above all, this innovative approach to home care seems to challenge all conventional wisdom and ingrained traditions and instill an inspiring sense of mission in its teams.

SWEDEN

Home help is the most frequently used service by the aged. It relies for the most part on part-time workers, mostly middle-aged women. It is hard to attract younger people, and to reverse this situation, some educational authorities have favored a social and health care orientation in technical high schools. Their hope that graduates from these high schools would eventually accept home care as a plausible career has not materialized, since only 4 percent of all home helpers are a product of these schools.

Home care workers would like to perform more social activities such as escorting, taking their patients outside for walks and to day-care programs, attending to their feelings of dejection and loneliness, and so forth, as distinguished from the more conventional tasks of cooking, housecleaning, and personal care.

This emerging role of friendly visitor, shaped around the image of a counselor or social worker, is more appealing to young high school graduates. It is also one that the district supervisors would specially like to emphasize. It would, however, require the creation of another layer of service to fill the remaining gaps, and municipalities claim they cannot afford it. For the moment, the friendly visitor role alone does not meet with some clients' most urgent needs and expectations. Moreover, some clients are fully satisfied with receiving just the home help services and rely on their relatives for the fulfillment of their social needs.

The proportion of elderly cared for by paid relatives has been steadily declining, from 25 percent of all home help workers in 1970 to 7 percent in 1986. In Stockholm, such care is reduced to only 1 percent. In nine out of ten cases the paid relative is a woman, usually in her forties, who does not work or works part-time outside her home. About 25 percent live with the person they care for, a phenomenon confined for the most part to rural areas.

Policymakers tend to resist the payment of relatives because they do not like the informality and alleged low professional standards involved in such arrangements. It must be borne in mind that most care is still provided by families who do not expect payment, as in the United States. Formal care is brought in either when there is no family available or when the relatives are incapable of assisting the person in need. The ratio of family members and home help workers generally overlap, and these care givers tend to coordinate their tasks informally.

Most of the home help service requirements are concentrated in the morning, from 7 to 11 A.M., and in the late afternoons, from 4 to 8 P.M.. It is difficult to organize a full-time working day or to divide it into two shifts, given this hourly spread. The service is also plagued by high absenteeism rates due to illness (mostly back problems), child care, and so forth.

Sweden has instituted liberal labor laws that authorize up to sixty days of paid leave a year. The net effect is that each municipality must ensure a steady flow of home help replacements. Many elderly resent it. They do not mind a constant rotation of new faces in the hospital, but they view things differently at home. They want to get used to the person upon whom they deposit their entire trust.

Home help services do offer workers attractive features: they pay wages comparable to the national average, they provide a certain independence and latitude in decision making, and they offer immediate gratifications. Most elderly clients do, after all, express their appreciation for the services they receive. The job is, however, physically and psychologically demanding, and it is not as socially valued as the more sophisticated technological occupations. Moreover, it is performed in conditions of relative isolation, without the presence or company of peers or supervisors. Some workers find this discouraging. It is not surprising, therefore, to find a high turnover rate, particularly among younger workers. They rarely last more than two years. Their main complaints are that they are locked in dead-end jobs without the prospect of climbing an enticing career ladder and that they have to work too many weekends. It must be recognized, however, that there is a small hard core that stays on the job for many more years. The staff turnover is not always due to resignations. It also results from systemic reorganizations, personnel rotations, and transfers.

Workers particularly complain of the physical aspects of the job, such as carrying bags and lifting handicapped persons to and from their beds, bathtubs, or toilets. True, they were specifically instructed to test whether patients can do any of these tasks by themselves. "You try first, and if you can't, I will give you a hand" is their standard invitation, resulting from the official self-help ideological framework. Many patients, however, become irate and retort that the home care worker is there "to do the things" for them, not to just watch them, keep them company, or tell them to take care of themselves.

The Swedish Association of Local Authorities (*Svenska Kommunforbundet*)—to which the 284 municipalities are affiliated—has observed that with unemployment reduced to a rate of 1.5 percent, adult women have been quickly incorporated into the private economic sector and no longer constitute the traditional pool from which municipalities drew their home helpers. This explains why they turned to the cohort of those 20 to 24 years of age, but as stated earlier, they have not yet found ways of retaining them for long. The turnover rate is 25 percent a year, but in some major urban centers like Stockholm, it reaches a 60 percent yearly rate. Salary improvements alone are not enough of an incentive to keep workers on the job. Home helpers, in fact, received the highest salary raises of all public-sector occupations in recent years. The association therefore proposed a three-tiered work load and job restructuring approach that encompasses the following:

1. Financial incentives to part-time workers who extend their work to a full seven-hour day. They would be paid for an extra hour, that is, eight hours' wages for seven hours of actual work.

2. More autonomy in organizing daily schedules.

3. Breaking the home help job into a wide range of career rungs, with the assurance of professionalization and predictable promotions.

Home health care is delivered by county visiting nurses in the counties' primary care offices. These nurses are for the most part practical nurses supervised by a licensed registered nurse.

Many municipalities pursue more systematic cooperation between the home help workers and the home nurses. The two services may thus schedule their work loads together rather than limiting their contacts to ad hoc conferences at the time of hospital discharge or initial client assessment. The home nurses then attend home help team meetings on a regular basis to review clients' progress and recommend new interventions.

It has been repeatedly observed that services occasionally tend to fall below standards due to inadequate supervision. Home help is also vulnerable at the midlevel of management. Municipal authorities consequently claim that there is a need for at least 50 percent more supervisors in order to iron out present service inconsistencies and overcome deficiencies.

All major political parties agree that the principle of normalization, that is, keeping the person at home, takes precedence over any other consideration of cost efficiency. Elected officials of both the Conservative and the Social Democratic parties concur in affirming this philosophical premise, but the Conservatives have misgivings about keeping home care services a virtual public monopoly. They favor instead privatization through a voucher system. While affirming that everybody is entitled to home care services, they would like to offer consumers a range of choices so that they can decide whom they want to have in their homes to assist them.

In order to introduce more service and manpower efficiency, a new law proposal was being framed at the time of this study aimed at subsuming all home care services, that is, home help and home health nursing, under the same authority. As stated earlier, these jobs are currently the responsibility of county councils and municipalities, respectively, which do not always see eye-to-eye on matters of fiscal jurisdiction.

ENGLAND

In England home nursing operates independently from its parallel home help service. Nurses are usually attached to a general practitioner or group of practitioners and work as part of a district nursing team. The nurses provide only health care, which may include supervising other health providers, monitoring quality of care, and negotiating for additional support services. Requests for an initial district nurse visit may be made by a general practitioner, a social service worker, the home help organizer, or the patient's family.

Throughout England, there has been a gradual trend towards improving the status of the home helps as the assistance they provide has shifted from purely domestic assignments to more personal care. As a consequence, they are now generally called "home care workers" rather than home helps. To some extent, this new status and title has facilitated recruitment.

In some areas of the country, such as in Hackney, a suburb of London, and Liverpool, the home helps have become unionized under a national agreement with the trade unions. This has guaranteed their benefits and also improved their pay structure. These factors combined with high rates of unemployment in these areas have actually resulted in a surplus of home helps. This, however, is not the case in London, where the employment rate is rather high and social service departments must compete with private industry for workers.

Most of the recruitment of home helps is done through local advertising and word-of-mouth. For part-time and nonunionized workers, the turnover rate can be as high as 40 percent annually. In some localities, workers are linked to clients who live in a specific geographic area and are thus restricted in their caseloads. If a client moves or dies, the worker can be left unemployed, a fact that contributes to insecurity and compounds the difficulties in retention.

England also has a well-established tradition of paying relatives. The attendants' allowances are paid directly to persons cared for at home who require assistance due to mental or physical disability. These persons can use this money to either purchase assistance privately or pay relatives for their services.

In addition, an invalid-care allowance is payable to persons under pensionable age if they look after a disabled person. The person must be caring for someone who qualifies and is deemed eligible to receive the attendance allowance, and the care giver must spend no less than thirty-five hours a week providing care. This category of paid family care-giver facilitates meeting the needs of a substantial number of dependent elderly.

England is one of the few countries that has set national guidelines for the training of home care workers. However, to date these guidelines refer only to the training of the home help organizers, that is, the supervisory ranks, and do not incorporate the paraprofessional workers.

A study made by the Social Services Inspectorate (Department of Health and Social Security, 1987) found that across the country the organizers in their roles as case managers exhibited no uniformity of practice, and often acted without reference to any formal standards. Moreover, their large caseloads, which averaged 210 per organizer, contributed to poorly organized case management.

The same study showed that in 1986 only 18.5 percent of these home help organizers had any relevant professional qualifications and that they lacked any systematic training. Such deficiencies contributed, according to the report, to ineffective service delivery, particularly in those increasingly complex cases involving frail elderly. These findings prompted the central government to allocate additional funds to the local governments for training the organizers. The availability of the funds is contingent on a minimum 30 percent local match. As evidence of the need for the program, the participation of local governments has actually exceeded the required minimum.

There are no established or uniform standards for the training of home help workers. Requirements, when they do exist, are set by the local governments and thus depend on local priorities and resources. Most home helps lack systematic training, a fact primarily due to budgetary limitations.

As an example, in Hackney, a borough of northeast London, workers must participate in an initial two-day training for which they receive regular compensation. They must then accompany experienced workers for several days and learn from their cases in the field. They receive a total of twelve full days of training from the local authority's social service department, during their first year of employment.

Liverpool offers an initial induction course of barely two hours, but the home helps then work for an entire week with an experienced worker. Every three months all home helps must participate in a two-week in-service training course, which is also delivered by the social service department.

The training requirements for home care nurses are, by contrast, fairly standardized throughout the country. These personnel are required to undergo basic hospital training as well as supplementary training in home nursing in a district office. This training is financed by the local health authorities, which require in exchange the commitment of at least one year of service.

THE NETHERLANDS

Home help or homemaking services are operated for the most part in a decentralized fashion, through district offices under the Central Council of Home Help. These offices are headed by a home help manager, usually a social worker, who supervises several teams of home helps. In 1988, Amsterdam had twelve such district offices, each staffed with two to three teams of ten home helps each.

In addition to directly managing the home help service, the district agencies also act as intermediaries between clients and a special type of paraprofessional, the "alpha helper." These are referred to clients who require between eight and twelve hours per week of domestic assistance but do not need any personal care. The alpha helpers are contracted directly by the clients, and the agency confines itself only to their recruitment and referral. Alpha helpers, consequently, are paid directly by the clients, who apply a specific government subsidy to this effect. The agency is not committed to cover the alpha's fringe benefits, since they operate as independent contractors.

The advantage of the alpha service to the home help agencies is that it allows them to concentrate on those cases requiring more intense care. The overall significance of the alpha helpers to home care is noted in the fact that in 1986 the Netherlands had approximately 40,000 alpha helpers and only 10,425 home helps.

The National Cross Association provides a vast array of services, including prenatal care, pregnancy classes, maternity care, health care for preschool children, and home nursing. However, 65 percent of their time is spent in home care. Moreover, 77 percent of the visits made by the nurses are to persons sixty years of age and older.

The main tasks performed by the nurses tend to exceed those usually associated with traditional nursing care. They may include health education, counseling, emotional support, and assistance in setting up informal support networks, as well as hospice care for dying patients and follow-up care for the families of patients who have died.

There are two professional categories of district nurses. The first requires four years of nursing education and an additional two years of experience in public health care. These nurses supervise the second level of paraprofessionals, who have had three years of hospital training and an additional six months in public health.

In some areas of the country there is an overabundance of first-level, or supervisory, nurses as compared to the second level of direct service practitioners. Shifting personnel, however, to make the service more cost-effective and reduce the number of supervisors is administratively cumbersome. The first-level nurses tend to resist any change in their job description that would require them to assume more direct services and force them to relinquish their supervisory roles.

Recruiting competent home helps is a difficult challenge in the highly urbanized areas of the Netherlands. Wages are set by the government but fall below the average levels of private industry. Moreover, in many areas home help agencies are competing for workers with independent providers who are paid directly by the clients. These workers receive approximately 20 percent more than agency counterparts. Efforts to attract more workers have included upgrading both the salary and the status of the home helps. To date, these attempts have had meager results, so in highly industrialized districts of Amsterdam, waiting lists of 150 persons for services are not uncommon.

Recruitment is done primarily through word-of-mouth and local advertising. Amsterdam has also tried giving bonuses to workers who recruit friends, but the shortage of workers persists. Young persons are often reluctant to work with the elderly arguing that they find it difficult to communicate with them. Agencies often recruit foreign immigrants to compensate for the shortage of personnel, but foreigners are frequently rejected by elderly clients on grounds of the inevitable language barriers.

A turnover rate of approximately 25 percent a year among the home helps is particularly felt in urban areas. The incidence is specially high in the first year of employment, but those who remain with the program for more than a year are likely to continue indefinitely. Special bonuses and recognition parties are strategies used to assist in retaining workers.

In addition, advanced training of home care workers facilitates status upgrading and better retention rates. More training leads to more responsibility and higher salaries. Home helps completing specialized courses are permitted to give injections and administer medications. Moreover, workers who obtain certificates in subjects such as "elder care" are also eligible for improved compensation.

Home helps in Amsterdam undergo sixteen hours of paid group training during their first three months of employment. They receive further training after one year on the job and are eligible for more specialized capacitation training after two or three years. This training is not conditional on a commitment to remain with the program. Regrettably, many do leave after completing the courses, attracted by the better-paying jobs in long term care institutions. The training curriculum covers a vast array of subjects, such as principles of social gerontology, psychological management of the elderly, health care, household management and upkeep, meals preparation and nutrition, recreation programs, and principles of rehabilitation.

MANITOBA, CANADA

The professionals operating the Continuing Care Program of Manitoba are nurses and social workers supported by two categories of paraprofessionals, the home attendants and the home care workers.

Manitoba's eight provincial regions are subdivided into district offices, which may further comprise rural substations. Each of these offices and substations is administered by a continuing-care coordinator, usually a social worker, in charge of planning, development, organization, and coordination. These tasks involve the data collection, monitoring, and review of all cases in the coordinator's jurisdiction. In some regions the coordinators also conduct assessments and home visits, although these are the primary responsibility of another category of professionals, the case coordinators.

Case coordinators are the actual case managers. They are either nurses or social workers, depending on the region. They assess patients, prepare their individual care plans, and assure the delivery of services that may include homemaking, physical therapy, occupational therapy, social work, and nursing. The case coordinators also represent their clients at the regional panels that determine whether a person requires nursing home placement.

Within each office, there is also a resource developer in charge of the recruitment, monitoring and evaluation of the homemakers, home attendants, and volunteers that constitute the nonprofessional staff of the home care service.

The nonprofessional staff in the Continuing Care Program consists of homemakers and home attendants. The primary role of the homemakers is to assist and monitor clients in their daily living tasks, including meal preparation, eating, taking medications set out by the nurse or primary care giver, cleaning the kitchen and bathroom, and doing the laundry. Specially trained homemakers may also assist the client with some personal care, bathing, and general hygiene. They are not authorized either to do shopping or to handle the client's money. They may, however, arrange for home delivery or for a neighbor to do the purchasing of needed items.

There are no special educational requirements for the homemakers, but they must have demonstrated competence in care giving. Most are middle-aged women with some background in institutional care. They do not get benefits other than the governmental Canadian pension plan, although they receive salary increments, holidays, and overtime. Home care workers are treated as casual employees, because very few work over thirty-five hours a week, and some work as little as three hours a week, the average being twenty-four hours. This ensures flexibility, but it also complicates the program's scheduling.

The home attendants focus on the personal care needs of the client. They assist with hygiene as well as coach the person to eat and to ambulate. They also assist with the elimination of body wastes in colostomy cases. In order to reduce duplication of tasks, attendants may also help with household maintenance and meal preparation, relieving the need for a homemaker.

Manitoba has less difficulty in recruiting home care workers than the European countries under review. There is generally no shortage of home helps, although it is somewhat more problematic to recruit in Winnipeg than in rural regions with higher rates of unemployment. The resource coordinator in each continuing-care office takes on the recruitment tasks. This is primarily done through talks to community groups and local advertising. These strategies generate sufficient numbers of applicants, although it is not easy to find workers for weekends and night shifts (8 P.M. to 8 A.M.).

Manitoba is one of the few areas where there is often a shortage of home care nurses. This occurs predominantly in the vast rural regions where there may be only one licensed practical nurse for a population of five thousand persons. The unsteady nature of the work makes it less appealing to registered nurses, who would rather have the employment stability and job security of an institution. The close social networks found in rural communities tend, however, to compensate for the nursing shortage. It is rare for a nurse to refuse taking on a case, since she usually knows the patient personally.

The Continuing Care Program provides the workers with some training, although according to program staff, it does not keep pace with the extent of need. The homemakers are trained one-half day a week for the first three to four months of work and receive regular wages while in training. There are also periodic in-service training sessions on special subjects such as dementia or incontinence. Homemakers completing additional special courses or training programs can move upward and become home attendants.

ARGENTINA

Home care services in Argentina are covered under the comprehensive national system of health care for the aged, which is administered by the federal Ministry of Social Action through its National Institute of Social Services for Retirees and Pensioners. More specifically, the services are provided directly by the Comprehensive Medical Care Program, PAMI. This program covers all persons sixty years of age and older. Eligibility is contingent on past contributions to the social security system or other public pension programs.

Only primary care physicians can submit a request for services to one of PAMI's district offices, where it is reviewed by both nursing and social work supervisors. The nurse supervisor subsequently draws a care plan, which may also include homemaking assistance. Home care services are available from 7 A.M. to 8 P.M. five days a week, but weekends are not covered.

Both home nursing and homemaker services are offered through the same district office of PAMI. The home nurse also teaches self-care education to the patient and the family. This may range from administering insulin injections to changing dressings. Nurse's aides provides the direct services, while registered nurses supervise, monitor, and review the status of the patients.

The homemakers, or domiciliary auxiliary workers, perform both personal and domestic tasks aimed at maintaining the person at home. They disinfect kitchens, beds, and bathrooms, take care of personal hygiene, help with dressing and ambulation, cook, feed if necessary, do laundry, and monitor medications. Their services extend outside the home to include shopping, banking, and paying bills. They encourage and assist their patients to perform some activities of daily living if they know of some residual capacity to do so.

Home nurses and domiciliary auxiliaries often work in teams, making joint visits to their patients. This is facilitated by the fact that they are both under the authority of the same district office.

The central factor in the national health system for the aged is the primary physicians, a cadre of private practitioners who sign part-time contracts for an assignment of five hundred to one thousand eligible older persons in a given district. Primary physicians are virtually case managers, authorizing and making referrals to other levels of services (hospitalization, nursing homes, outpatient specialists) and home care. Also, the physician is expected to make home visits, when needed.

In recent years, due to Argentina's large foreign debt and trade deficit and its escalating rate of inflation, there has been a curtailment of the budgets for health and social services. This has resulted in many of the voluntary nonprofit agencies developing their own innovative programs involving home care workers.

The Jewish Welfare Association, as an example, recruits, trains, and places homemakers but does not hire them. Instead, it subsidizes elderly clients so that they can enter into a private contractual agreement with a homemaker. The task of recruiting homemakers usually falls to the social worker assigned to the specific case. The social worker begins by canvassing the neighborhood or asking the client's acquaintances if they would be willing to assist the person for a paid hourly fee. The Jewish Welfare Association does not maintain a roster of home helps. Recruitment is consequently a continual process.

The Municipality of Buenos Aires

The city of Buenos Aires decided it was imperative to step in and fill the home care service gaps left by the federal government. It realized that there were too many elderly who had never worked and did not qualify for social security and related benefits and who, consequently, could not apply for PAMI's home care services. In addition, it wished to create a home care program that took into consideration the person's social needs and transcended the narrowly defined medical model utilized by PAMI.

The city's program is in its incipient stages. It took two years to plan, and a great deal of care went into both the training curriculum and the criteria for selecting the trainees, who will be designated upon graduation as "geriatric auxiliaries." The program's most remarkable feature, at this point, is perhaps the painstaking sophistication of its training model. Among the program's intended features are the following:

1. *Eligibility.* Elderly persons over sixty will be able to apply directly, without a medical referral. They will have to meet only three eligibility requirements: they must be sixty years of age or older; they must not be covered by the federal program or must lack adequate income; and they must be self-sufficient in the activities of daily living or experience only a moderate degree of dependence. The last requirement basically means that applicants must be able to get in and out of bed by themselves, move around the house, and feed themselves without help. In cases of moderate dependency, a designated relative will be responsible for the continuity of care when the geriatric auxiliary is not present.

2. *Definition of services.* Home care services will include personal hygiene and grooming; meals preparation; medication administration (only oral and when medically prescribed); laundry, including ironing and mending; homemaking in the entire dwelling if the person lives alone, or in the bedroom only if the client lives with a relative; shopping for medications and food; escorting the person to medical appointments and to collect benefits; keeping company at home; essential physical rehabilitation tasks, such as walking or light exercises prescribed by a rehabilitation center; and recreational and occupational activities, including suggestions of television programs, readings in newspapers and magazines, and arts and crafts. The home attendant or geriatric auxiliary will facilitate the client's getting out into the community and participating in meetings, group activities, parties, artistic performances, and so on.

   The main philosophical thrust of the city's home care service is social integration and community participation. It consequently aims to focus on relatively well-functioning or moderately impaired older persons who are at risk of becoming isolates. The program is therefore conceived as social support and makes no pretense of including any intensive nursing or convalescent treatment component.

3. *Funding.* Service users will receive a municipal subsidy to cover the home care costs. This allowance will be graduated in relation to the user's actual income and resources. Social workers will assess each applicant's capacity to pay. The municipal subsidy or allowance will be limited to the hourly wages for the geriatric auxiliaries. The total monthly allowance may not exceed 70 percent of the cost for the full institutionalization in any of the municipal homes for the aged. The program will be entirely funded with municipal revenues.

4. *Employment.* The city will not be the ultimate employer of the geriatric auxiliaries, even if it does recruit, screen and train them. Instead, city authorities are considering incorporating them as a service cooperative, to be run and administered by the workers themselves.

5. *Administration.* The home care program will be directed by a coordinator, assisted by a technical team, and will report to the city's General Administration of Social Services. Requests for services and referrals will be lodged at the municipal social services district offices. Social workers at the district offices will assess each application and determine whether it qualifies for service. They will in turn refer the documentation with their recommendation for a specific and individualized service plan to the central coordinator's office. It is at this level only that decisions will ultimately be made. Authorizations will therefore be entirely centralized. The entire process, however, may not take more than fifteen days before a request for services is granted or denied.

6. *Duration of services.* Services will be time-limited and may not exceed a six-month period. A new cycle of service, however, may be authorized if the city district social workers make a recommendation to this effect.

7. *Quality of care.* Both the city district social workers and the central coordinator's office will monitor the quality of the services delivered and determine whether they meet formal standards. They will conduct meetings to this effect with service users, their families, and the home attendants.

8. *Manpower training.* The municipality of Buenos Aires is offering an intensive program of training to future home attendants. It consists of six hours of formal class contact a week for four months, plus daily group discussion sessions. Each group consists of twelve students and is led by a district social worker. The groups link class conceptual information to practical cases and issues.
   The curriculum covers subject areas such as social gerontology, psychological management of elderly clients, health issues, household management and upkeep, meals preparation and nutrition, recreation programs, and principles of rehabilitation.

The municipal program was conceived as an alternative to the highly medicalized service model operated by the federal government. Its intent is to promote the elderly clients' self-sufficiency and to link them to recreational and socialization programs in order to overcome the risks of depression and isolation. It underscores a social orientation that involves the family and connects the client to his or her immediate community. Its uniqueness also rests on the recreation and occupational therapy components usually found only in senior centers. It is as if the home attendant first brings the senior center into the client's home, and then proceeds to escort the client to the senior center. This is indeed a specialized program geared to the well aged who are at risk of isolation. It does not tackle the problems of multiple chronicity and convalescence of the more frail elderly.

CONCLUSION

All countries distinguish between home health or home nursing services on the one hand, and home help or homemakers' functions on the other. These domains tend, however, to overlap. Homemakers are increasingly assigned paraprofessional nursing, occupational therapy, or social work tasks. This modicum of role integration is meant to neutralize the worker's boredom and to attend to the client as a whole person. There are also efficiency considerations, since the integration may also reduce the need for or the quantity of routine home nursing visits. It is usually claimed that the trend towards role blurring implies for the most part an upgrading of the homemaker rather than a downgrading of the nurse and/ or home nurse.

A further specialization within the ranks of homemakers points out the difference between the above-mentioned generalists who attend to most basic activities of daily living and environmental upkeep and the heavy-duty or basic specialists who wash floors, windows, and bathrooms, move furniture, and carry heavy household or health equipment. The most common model is one in which a national health insurance program or a similar public welfare fund subsidizes consumers so that they may hire directly the heavy-duty contractors.

Staff is often recruited among middle-aged women, students, and even elderly retirees seeking part-time work. Relatives and neighbors may be specially targeted if they live with the patient or nearby. The advantage of employing relatives is a greater sense of commitment as well as the possibility that they may be willing to extend their services to other persons in need in their immediate vicinity.

The recruitment of relatives is, however, the strategy of last resort. This strategy is based upon the fact that turnover rates of home care workers is very high and that consequently it is not worthwhile to invest too much in their training. It recognizes the unskilled and lower status of home care in an occupational market dominated by more upwardly mobile and more high-tech service professions. Finally, it accepts that the high turnover rates will continue, and consequently it will emphasize aggressive outreach and recruitment at the local or district levels rather than training and retention.

An opposite, more professionally oriented, recent model seeks to upgrade the status of home care in its diverse modalities by instituting lengthier training, better pay, full-time employment, periodic retraining, counseling and support services, attractive health and pension benefits, and the semblance of a career ladder. A major liability, however, is that more professional home care workers may emphasize the social and therapeutic side of their tasks to the detriment of the more basic household tasks.

Most countries are heavily invested in testing new retention strategies. Some of these include paid travel time, paid training time, clothing allowances, health leave days, psychological counseling and consultation; paid group support time, full fringe benefits for part-time employment, team rather than solo visits to clients' homes, team planning and rotation in household tasks, rotation between household and nursing home or senior-center duties, greater discretion and participation in services planning, and ratios of one hour of education for every three hours of direct service, among others. The extent of success of these strategies remains limited, given the continuing high turnover rate of home care personnel.

6

Innovative Programs: Organizational Demonstrations

This study was specially aimed at highlighting new trends in home care services. It was observed that some of the innovations involve a more comprehensive restructuring of the operational framework of service delivery, while others focused more heavily on the manpower component.

This chapter deals with the first type, that is, programs known for having reconceptualized the very purpose of home care. For the most part, they have also redefined both the meaning of the long-term care continuum and the linkages of home care with other critical services for the frail and homebound, such as nursing home care, congregate housing, and day care. In each instance, they have embarked in significant organizational and administrative departures from the standardized models prevailing in their countries.

THE DRAMMEN EXPERIMENT

Drammen is a midsized municipality located 45 km south of Oslo. It has lost most of its industrial base but is now developing a thriving service economy. The town has a long-standing home care tradition that dates back to the 1920s. In fact, the first official public home care service in Norway seems to have started in Drammen. It originally consisted of two or three nurses visiting private domiciles in search of homebound and frail persons. By 1985, Drammen realized that while the organization had developed a solid grass-roots tradition and a viable operational infrastructure, it was lacking the coordinative functions essential to a strong organization. The municipality was then divided into six districts, each directed by a head nurse. Drammen gradually developed a work force of over seven hundred home helpers, although only a fifth of them were full-time, salaried workers at the time of this study.

Drammen's home care model hinges on the systematic reduction of beds and a new philosophy about the role of the nursing home as an institution. The municipal authorities are engaged in a three-year plan to reduce the number of nursing home beds by 25 percent, from 521 to 399, or from a rate of 8.6 to 6.5 per hundred elderly. Because the nursing homes are under the same municipal authority as the home care services, the savings obtained from the reduction will be applied to an expansion of home care services, including intensive round-the-clock home health nursing. This policy reflects an ideological aversion to institutional care and, conversely, a concerted effort to keep patients at home as the ultimate criterion of program success. Even those who can no longer remain at home will be housed in congregate residences supported by a heavy infusion of home help and home nursing services.

Given the philosophical conviction that continuity of life style and quality of life are the foremost objectives, cost-efficiency considerations become secondary. The city's health care authority may even provide income supports for paying the rental of a patient's permanent dwelling while he or she is placed in a congregate housing facility. The expectation in all instances is that patients will return to their original homes. Given this type of health care model, it is not surprising that whenever nursing home care is prescribed, it is only for short-term, rehabilitative purposes.

Each of the six district leaders has the authority to decide how and where placement of a client will take place and how much home nursing, home help, or nursing home care should be offered. All decisions rest on an initial standardized battery of evaluative instruments similar to those used in other parts of the country. However, in designing individual care packages, greater emphasis is placed on staff conferences and intensive daily consultations with all service providers.

District leaders work in daily contact with hospitals and obtain from them the lists of admissions that originate in their own jurisdictions. They then contact the patient and the family to ascertain the home arrangements and services needed at the time of discharge. The leaders oversee the discharge process, and while the patient is still in the hospital, they conduct a home visit to determine the suitability of the home environment. The leaders may recommend a number of possible physical adjustments, such as hand bars and bathtub nonskidding mats, a new bed, or even an elevator. They may also require prosthetic and safety devices, such as "emergency buzzers" or "lifelines" that patients wear around their necks, and a closer monitoring by the district fire station of those elderly who are especially vulnerable because of a recent hospitalization.

Hospitals have the sole authority of discharging patients, even though the district leader assumes the coordinating task of planning the discharge. Given that hospitals tend to discharge as soon as possible, the home care staff may advocate a longer stay in the hospital if all environmental adjustments and required services are not yet in place. Hospitals, for the most part, do not challenge these requests and will agree to a later discharge, even if it means incurring greater costs.

Each district receives a fixed budget to cover the costs of institutional care, home care, day care, cash supports, rental subsidies, congregate meals, and administrative overhead. Each is also allocated funds to buy apartments for housing mild Alzheimer's cases. These housing units are linked in a communal arrangement that facilitates the provision of home and congregate services. For those suffering a more advanced stage of the disease, separate units in nursing homes have been instituted.

Funding requests by the districts are the outcome of exhaustive reviews of needs by nursing home directors and district leaders. Even though the elderly population leveled off in numbers, Drammen has been experiencing an increase in services costs of 7 percent a year due to the demand for more intensive levels of care. The budget is based on an overall yearly projection of 300,000 home help hours or units of service and 50,000 hours of home nursing care. An old policy established a maximum of 15 hours of home help a week per client. Home nursing visits were limited to four times a day, with a maximum of one and a half hours per visit.

These limits, however, were replaced by a more flexible criterion: patients needing more attention receive it, on a case-by-case basis. The average amount of hours for home help is three hours a week. The Drammen authorities do not agree, however, with the criterion adopted in other parts of the country that says if a client needs more than 6.5 hours a week of services it is more economical to resort to an institutional solution, since such need may be exceptional and last for only a short period.

Drammen's municipal budget for services is reinforced with block grants received from the central government. All home care recipients, however, are required to pay a membership fee to the municipality, similar to a prepaid registration to a health maintenance organization in the United States. All participants pay the same fee regardless of the number of units of service they receive. The fee is established on a sliding scale basis, from a maximum of 190 kroner a month (about $35, at the time the study was conducted) to no charge at all. Since the municipal health authority can access all individual income tax returns, it can immediately determine the corresponding fee for each beneficiary. A similar sliding formula is applied to nursing home users, who can be charged no more than 16,000 kroner a month, or $2,952. This latter amount applies, however, to those with incomes of 250,000 kroner (or $46,000). Most older persons receive the minimum yearly pension of 50,000 kroner, ($9,225) and are required to pay approximately 2,917 kroner ($538) a month for nursing home care. If families cannot afford the services charged to an elderly relative, they may be enlisted to provide some of the home help themselves and receive compensation for up to four hours per week. The municipality benefits substantially from this arrangement because the professional home care staff is then freed to attend to other emergencies.

Home helpers visit their assigned patients in teams of up to seven workers each. Each district operates several such units. The teams meet each morning to review each client's status, plan services, and decide who should be placed on the priority list. Team members are guaranteed permanency in their jobs and have no need, therefore, to inflate or exaggerate the severity of their clients' conditions. This used to be prevalent when home helpers worked alone. They would often postpone reporting on a client's improvement or minimize it, for fear of losing a steady flow of income. It is also hoped that the team approach will reduce the loneliness and stress experienced by individual workers and thus reduce the burnout syndrome.

THE VANG EXPERIMENT

Vang is a small commune of 1,700 people perched in the central mountains northeast of Oslo and halfway between the capital city and the western coast of fjords. Vang is atypical because its proportion of elderly residents is 50 percent higher than the national average. The capital city, Oslo, by contrast exceeds that average by only 7 percent. The municipality experienced a dramatic increase in the demand for geriatric services by elderly persons who were left behind when their children moved to urban areas.

Until 1983, the town followed the classical model of services that separated health from social services. It was proud of its "red" building, as residents commonly referred to the "hospital for people who cannot live alone," but its complacency was shattered when the twenty-six-bed hospital, actually a nursing home, reached capacity and had no more beds available. There were no home care services to handle the overflow. The average length of stay per patient was then 125 weeks, and the commune authorities realized that it was becoming a form of permanent residence.

Searching for solutions, they began with a defined philosophy of services that encompassed the following principles:

1. Services will be given to all those who request them, on a non-declining basis. All those who need services will receive them without delay. Consequently, there will be no waiting lists.
2. The staff must visit patients in their homes.
3. Health and social services will be consolidated into a single comprehensive service.
4. There will be no limits to the provision of services: if a person needs home care 365 days per year, it will be available on a nondeclining basis.

The Vang authorities also deemed that for each patient there would be a comprehensive care plan that would outline and record all services and assigned personnel. Copies of this care plan and records were to be shared with the head nurse, the home help worker, the patient and all informal supports, such as family who were part of the care plan. In 1987, four years after the Vang experiment began, authorities claimed to have reduced the nursing home average length of stay to forty-three weeks, or about one-third. The monies saved were applied to enhancing home care services, which increased from about one thousand units of service to four thousand. The most important feature, however, is that institutional care and home care are no longer dichotomous but are interchangeable services, linked by the assignment of the same workers to both, thus minimizing paperwork, referrals and case conferences.

The operational model is as follows: The commune is divided into four districts. Each has a primary nurse or district leader who works two days in the district making home visits. The leader then spends the remaining three days in the nursing home following home care patients, most of whom alternate between their homes and the institution. In addition, the leader acts as a de facto case manager who provides the continuity of care for each patient.

Most patients spend one day a week as residents of the nursing home. They come for regular checkups, physiotherapy, occupational therapy, rehabilitation, nutrition, or just to socialize with other people of their district. For most of them the institution serves as a senior center, day-care program, and rehabilitation and treatment center. They are brought by cab, a service arranged by the municipality, but they can come only on the days when their primary nurses are doing their tour of duty in the nursing home. All programmatic distinctions give way to a client-centered, integrated model.

Ambulatory patients living alone are required to use the lifeline device in order to alert the nursing home and hospital of any emergencies. The Vang authorities are aware of the similarities between their model and that of Drammen, but point out that the latter is more expensive because it separates home care and nursing home care as distinct services. The Vang model is cheaper, they claim, because it does not accept that distinction.

A good system, they finally add, is one in which people do not have to wait for services. Waiting lists generate uncertainty and make people anxious, causing them to place themselves on the lists even if they do not need the services with any urgency. The service practice in Vang is designated with three T's—*Tillit, Trivsel, Trygghet,* which means trust, well-being, and safety. It reflects the assurance that the elderly can trust the system and will receive a home nurse or home helper without delay.

The Vang model does not preclude that families and volunteers ought to play a substantial role. The municipality runs a campaign to educate the community at large, through its nearly fifty voluntary organizations. The post office and shopkeepers are on the alert for any symptoms of bizarre behavior, long absences, and sudden frailty. This modality of relentless outreach rests on the informal social networks that facilitate the early detection of many problems.

Once a referral is made, the district nurse visits the person and conducts a psychosocial assessment. It is noteworthy that the nurse assumes a role usually reserved in most other countries for the social worker. The municipality does employ social workers, but they are assigned to broader social problem areas such as alcoholism, child abuse, family conflict, and, more recently, drug addiction and refugees.

Aging is the sole domain of nursing, which also exercises the administrative authority over its contingent of home help workers. The district nurse works out the plan of services for each case and assigns a limited number of hours of home nurse and/or home help care.

Home health care workers are organized in teams responsible for all the aging population in their defined geographical domain. Each team organizes its schedules and relates to other professionals through their group leader. The team decides when to invite the contact nurse to their meetings, although either this nurse or the team can take the initiative to this effect. Vang has given primacy to an autonomous paraprofessional team model, a substantial departure from most Norwegian municipal approaches, which center around a professional nurse.

Home care services are not free. Charges hinge on each person's ability to pay. Confidentiality is apparently not a major concern in small rural localities like Vang. Through bank and tax records, the Department of Health and Social Services is able to determine the financial resources of each client. The standard charge is ten kroner ($1.85) per visit, and only 10 percent of the aged are unable to pay. On the whole, the municipality provides about one thousand free units of home care services each year, or 25 percent of the total.

Contrary to the situation in larger urban areas, there is no shortage of home helpers in Vang. Most of the part-time home care workers are farm women, and each works between five and ten hours per week. At the time of the study there were forty part-timers, with a work-load equivalency of seven full-time staff members. The municipality refuses to hire too many full-time workers because it is believed that they become too professionalized, and unionized, and thus, become prisoners of self-imposed restrictions that destroy the personal relationship and the continuity of contact with each patient's social networks. The municipality prefers to receive recommendations for new staff from the elderly themselves or their social networks. Ideally, the municipality would like to have one home helper for each cluster of blocks or sectors in the district.

Norwegian law does not require that part-time workers employed less than ten hours a week be accorded benefits. However, the municipality extended benefits to this group voluntarily as a means of enhancing the workers' sense of occupational value and providing an incentive to stay in the service.

Home helpers come as close as possible to becoming surrogate family members, and confidants. Older persons reveal to them most of their intimate apprehensions and thoughts. This puts an unfair discretionary burden on the home helpers, as they are often unsure when to follow the rules of confidentiality and when to report a new situation. The municipality has decided to withstand that risk, since it is nearly impossible to determine how to proceed in each case, and it is most important to maintain the informal quality of the relationship.

Moreover, the municipal Department of Health and Social Services observed that older persons do not particularly care if the home nurse changes frequently, but they insist upon the same home helper. They consider the first a professional and the second, a personal friend. Because of the role home helps play in the social universe of their aging clients, the municipality decided that these workers will not perform hands-on services, such as bathing, cutting toenails, and the like. These tasks are reserved for the home nurse. The home helpers, on the other hand, perform the chore services in the house.

THE SANDEFJORD'S SENIOR-CENTER MODEL

Sandefjord is an old whaling port of thirty-seven thousand inhabitants about 90 kilometers southeast of Oslo. Like Drammen, its neighbor to the north, it is attempting to shape a viable system of services for its five thousand senior citizens.

This system is based on the premises that home care should function as follows:

1. Gradually replace rather than complement nursing home care.
2. Include a rehabilitation orientation, not mere supportive care.
3. Invest in community based, senior-center programming as an essential service component.
4. Use discretion concerning the extent to which families and relatives will participate in the care plan. Some families may be a hindrance more than effective rehabilitation agents.
5. Treat the entire person, not a specific disability, and also attend to the person's interests, not only his or her needs.

The objective is to have older, frail persons continue as "responsible adults" and not succumb to despondency and dependency. To this effect, home care workers encourage them to do as much as possible for themselves. Home care personnel are trained precisely to start out as "trainers" capable of detecting their clients' remaining potentialities and strengths and to motivate them to assume as much self-care as possible. Of course, this is not applicable to all clients. Many have little or no rehabilitation potential left, as in the case of terminally ill, dying, or mentally incompetent patients.

Sandefjord does not prescribe conventional nursing home care in all terminal cases, due to its open-care model. Terminal patients may die in their own homes, if desired, and are tended with intensive nursing. They are housed in specifically renovated community retirement flats. This arrangement is parenthetically related to the American concept of congregate living, but it does not involve separate, specially designated facilities. The municipality acquires clusters of apartments in regular residential buildings where the elderly and disabled are integrated with people of all ages. They retain there a sense of normal living and privacy, but receive varying degrees of home health and home help supports. Furthermore, they are constantly monitored through a triple system of alarms, emergency telephones, and lifeline bracelets. These buildings are close to one of the five municipal district offices where the district nurses and their home care personnel are based. Any of these workers can be alerted to an emergency in a matter of minutes, if not seconds. Additional innovations are the "night patrols," or teams of home health workers and home helpers that follow up patients with special problems and those who are convalescing after a recent hospitalization.

These home care workers visit up to five times a day, if needed, regardless of whether the total costs exceed those of comparable nursing home care. In these circumstances the service system seeks to establish an active partnership with all potential informal supports—relatives, friends, and neighbors—and jointly plan a schedule of care.

The more traditional and medically oriented nursing homes have not been entirely abandoned, even though Sandefjord has vowed not to build new ones. The town has divided the current stock of 287 beds into two systems, short-term care, or STC, and the better-known long-term care (LTC). The STC comprises 30 beds, plus 20 earmarked for strict rehabilitation purposes. Their use is limited to a three-week maximum. LTC totals, in turn, 167 beds, which cannot be used for more than six months, although this upper limit is rather flexible.

While it has become harder to get into a nursing home, there are no universal guidelines prescribing who will be admitted. The decision rests on an exchange between the district leader, the local doctor, the family, and the home nursing personnel involved in the case. There are three local medical practitioners in each district, and each is assigned a special telephone to be used only for consultation in cases requiring home care or institutionalization. This arrangement ensures that physicians are effective members of the decision-making team. They are required, in fact, to reserve several hours a week for review and consultation regarding difficult cases.

The reduction and freeze in the number of nursing home beds clashed with the reality of lengthy waiting lists. These, however, were gradually reduced through a meticulous process of one-on-one counseling with applicants. It was found that many only needed reassurance that they would receive care, having applied for an entire gamut of services just to be safe.

In these cases, STC was recommended, with specific treatment goals agreed upon with the applicant. At the end of the three-week period, the staff would assess what had been accomplished. This STC period operates on the basis of contracts for functional rehabilitation, and it may be eventually extended if new rehabilitative objectives are identified and agreed upon. Service applicants are reassured they are being taken care of and that the system is attentive to their needs.

The system in question is available to all community residents and does not require professional referrals. District leaders visit each applicant, assess each one's condition, and check to see if there is a functional primary support network. The district leader often finds out that the family is not aware of the applicant's needs, simply because the latter does not wish to bother them. The opposite may also be the case: the district leader may observe that the family exercises a deleterious effect on the patient, usually in the form of an overprotective attitude that fosters dependence and excess disability. In these instances the district nurse may judge that some distance between generations is needed and suggest that the family limit its involvement. All first contacts eventually lead to a contract that spells out what will be done in the first week or month and by whom. The district staff will conduct the reevaluation at the end of the agreed-upon time period and recommend what, if any, additional assistance is required.

As in most of Norway, securing a reliable home care work force proved to be a major hurdle for the Sandefjord municipal authorities. In 1987, 30 percent of the vacancies remained unfilled. This operational deficit was soon remedied by means of a new salary scale that not only exceeded the national norm but also was much higher than that of the more prestigious hospitals and nursing homes. Municipal planners believe, however, that this was only part of the story. They attribute a good measure of their success to a philosophy of care that involves clients in their own care and views them as total persons, not just as disease entities occupying hospital beds. This new perception proved to be very appealing to many nurses and nurse's aides searching for a more community-oriented type of work.

The most original feature of the Sandefjord program is, indeed, the active role performed by the senior center within the long-term care system. Most of the one thousand senior-center members are self-sufficient and independent, "well" aged. The senior center and personal home care services complement each other through a system of mutual referrals. The center's programming is intended to foster a higher level of self-directed activities, which may prevent or limit the need for home care services. Such programming is built around the notion or concept of like-minded networks, that is, people who share the same interests and actively pursue them together.

Each network establishes its internal routines, and its members—not the staff—can easily ascertain if another member falls behind, no longer participates, or is having problems. Networks may then speak to or counsel the member and determine whether the problem is transitory or whether it requires professional inputs. Each network thus acts as an early detection and warning system. The center houses about seventy to seventy-five such networks, also referred to as clubs or peer systems, all of which are self-organized and self-directed. The center staff is occasionally invited to attend some of the clubs' meetings or activities, but plays a minor role in their governance and operation. Concurrent with this interdependence between senior-center and long-term care services, the staff asks all new members during the initial interview whether they live alone, who takes care of them, whether they need help at home, and what their interests and life experiences are.

The senior center places great philosophical emphasis on two principles:

1. It does not accept volunteerism on the part of its members as a form of donation or charity. It will accept their work contribution, however, under a formal agreement or contract, provided it is consistent with the center's interests.

2. It will facilitate programs that enhance continuity of lifelong

interests. As an example, one network was made up of former boaters wishing to practice their sport. The center rented a boat and paid for it from its regular budget.

The center cannot offer empirical proof that its emphasis on interest-focused peer networks actually neutralizes the onset of frailty and dependence. It does, however, provide evidence that the members who are well actively incorporate the moderately frail members in their social and activity programs. It is conceivable that the emphasis on peer support lessens the risks of or postpones loneliness and depression as well as the internalization of a "helpless" attitude that often precedes the virtual state of dependence. There is no empirical evidence, however, to prove it.

THE TABY EXPERIENCE

Taby is a modern and prosperous municipality of 55,000 people located on the outskirts of Stockholm. The population sixty-five years of age and older numbers six thousand, or 11 percent, a proportion substantially below the national average. The demographic predominance of the young is reflected in the municipal home care caseload. Besides the frail elderly, it includes a higher than average number of young handicapped and victims of severe accidents, terminally ill persons, and substance abusers.

Taby's model of home care services reflects, for the most part, the same standard version implemented all over Sweden. There are, however, operational nuances and differences of emphasis that stem from local social and political circumstances as well as the community's persistent ingenuity. It is worth highlighting the most important differences as an example of municipality planning:

1. Home helpers take greater than average responsibility for personal care. The most frequent tasks are bathing, washing and setting hair, and cutting nails. They also administer insulin injections, change wound dressings, monitor the intake of prescribed medications, and assist with the person's functional mobility and activities of daily living. For the latter, a general orientation to the basics of physical therapy is included in their basic training.

2. Food preparation and feeding is a similarly dominant occupational agenda. Home helpers may bring hot meals prepared in the kitchens of service houses, warm up frozen meals, or cook.

3. Clients are assigned to rotating teams of four to five home help-

ers, which means they do not have to depend on a single worker but become familiar with the entire team. This shared-assistance concept circumvents the problems of absenteeism, sickness, or vacations, since there is no need for temporary replacements or stand-ins.

4. Full-time home helpers take care of four to five clients a day. The day is divided into task-related periods. Generally speaking, personnel care services are reserved for the early morning and late afternoon. More specifically, the first period includes breakfast preparation, bathing, and dressing. The second, in midmorning, is for shopping, errands, and cleaning. The third, around noon, is for bringing or preparing lunch and cleaning, and the fourth, in early afternoon, is for cleaning, errands, and escorting to doctors' offices. The team arranges its daily and weekly schedules according to the client's most pressing needs and in a way that distributes the physical load equitably among the workers.

5. Similarly to other municipalities, home helpers work with both clients living in the community and those residing in service houses. They can work with only one group if they so choose. At times this creates logistics problems, but it is accepted in order to enhance the staff's sense of initiative and morale.

6. Initial training is limited to one to two weeks, most of it accompanying an experienced home help worker in the field. Training continues, however, in an intermittent but consistent way. Workers receive one to two additional weeks each year, parceled out in short, intensive seminars about issues such as acting-out behavior, psychiatric disorders, care of the terminally ill patient, developmental disabilities, and so forth. In addition, workers receive continuous consultation and psychological support from a backup team of psychiatrists, psychologists, and social workers. The issues brought to these professionals by individual workers may be selected as the topic for a teamwide seminar.

7. Taby is particularly proud of the level of cooperation it has achieved between the municipal home helpers and the county home nurses. Rather than limiting themselves to ad hoc contacts at the time of hospital discharge and initial assessment, the two branches of home care share the ongoing services process by scheduling their work together. Home nurses attend the home helpers' meetings to review clients' progress, hear home helpers' reports about emerging problems, and recommend new interventions.

Taby's municipality authorities are aware, however, that as the number of both disabled and very old residents keeps increasing, the local home care services will not be able to cope with the demand for services. They therefore claim that home care must be supplemented by a parallel and extensive network of day-care services, a position that carries considerable weight on municipal planning agendas. The interface between day care and home care constitutes the next challenge and the inevitable wave of the future.

THE NÖRKOPING EXPERIENCE

Nörkoping, one of Sweden's largest cities, is located about 100 miles southwest of Stockholm. It was a major textile center in the past, but today it boasts having a more diversified industrial base, and is home for the headquarters of some of the country's largest electronics corporations.

The city's home care services evolved within the context of an ecological model aimed primarily at modernizing the housing stock. The ensuing urban renewal process proceeded hand-in-hand with parallel improvements in the social services. The coordination between the two was considered essential for the creation of a better and stronger sense of community identity.

The process of environmental modernization initiated by the municipality was guided by the following objectives:

1. The provision of a higher standard of housing.
2. The integration of people of different social backgrounds and ages.
3. The belief that older and handicapped people should be able to stay in their own homes.
4. The participation of residents in decisions affecting their immediate environment.

In order to implement those objectives, a three-pronged redevelopment strategy was initiated. First, old but structurally sound neighborhood housing projects were gutted and rebuilt to suit contemporary requirements. Some apartments were specially fitted with prosthetic devices and altered for the convenience of frail and handicapped persons. Access was specially improved, with the installation of elevators in all the four-storied buildings.

Second came the installation of a series of services such as (1) community centers with meals for the elderly, to be operated by the local residents on a cooperative basis; (2) day-care centers for the handicapped;

(3) the stationing of home nursing and medical personnel from both municipal and county services on the premises of each housing complex; and (4) retirees' support groups and clubs for both the well and the frail.

The third approach entailed the integration of home care services within the total ecological strategy and, most specially, with day care. Municipal planners hypothesized that once all the above-mentioned environmental supports and improvements in the quality of life were in place, the demand for home help would eventually decline. The municipality has moved away from the service house concept prevalent in the country at large and begun experimenting with small-group living, especially for the demented elderly. This entails consolidating five to six apartments in each residential complex into a service unit that may receive round-the-clock home help and home nursing services. These are calibrated not only according to each resident's needs, but also by taking into account if there are well-functioning spouses capable of assisting with at least some of the activities of daily living. Furthermore, the group-living residents are transported by taxis—the cost is subsidized through a voucher system—to a day-care center where they spend eight hours daily, seven days a week. The meals, stimulation, and personal and nursing care they receive at the center substantially reduce the volume of services they might otherwise require at home.

Home help and home nursing care services in Nörkoping follow, for the most part, the organizational and operational models found in other communities. As in Taby, special incentives aimed at enhancing worker morale and efficiency have been added. Home helpers are thus periodically rotated among individual homes, group residences, day centers, and even retirees' club (where they help with meals and activities) in order to introduce a measure of variety in their jobs. They also work in teams of two when dealing with the very sick or handicapped. The two workers alternate the heavy and lighter tasks, such as household chores and social stimulation. The local authorities have combined one hour of paid education for every three hours of work in order to increase the job's attractiveness and facilitate the recruitment of new personnel.

It is not surprising that the preceding selection includes programs in Norway and Sweden. The decentralized governmental system in these two countries, coupled with a minimum of regulatory controls, creates a favorable environment for creative planning initiatives.

7

Innovative Programs: Utilization of Manpower Resources

This chapter continues the selective inventory of innovative programs. While the preceding chapter highlighted several creative departures in the conceptual and operational domains, the present one examines emerging new manpower strategies. The recruitment, retention, and supervision of home care workers is a major concern in most of the countries included in this study. The following cases illustrate how specific programs cope with the limited availability of human resources and seek, at the same time, to improve the quality of the services they deliver.

KENT

Kent is a large and relatively affluent county in the southeast of England. Its three-year plan, detailed in *Services for the Elderly in Kent: Planning for the Future*, was adopted by the county council in 1987. Among its distinctive features are increases in short-term residential and respite care, day-care placements, and increased support to informal care givers. These services exceed those customarily provided by the traditional home help programs and social service departments.

There are thirty-two community care schemes, or programs, across the county. These were initiated in the midseventies with the aim of coordinating community care for those frail elderly who would otherwise require institutional care. Each scheme is based upon a community care organizer, similar to a case manager, who undertakes the coordination of all of the services needed by each client and the liaison with the agencies.

Organizers are assigned relatively small caseloads so that they can become better acquainted with their clients and blend resources more effectively. Each client is allocated an individual budget from which the organizer purchases services. However, expenditures on individual cases are limited to two-thirds the equivalent monthly cost of a bed in a residential home.

Dartford's Community Care Program

Dartford is one of the largest cities in Kent. Its community care program has been in existence since 1983. The program is administered by a principal social worker for elderly care and is under the direct supervision of a community care organizer. The community care team includes the organizer, two community care assistants, three home help organizers, two social workers, a social work assistant, and a worker for the visually handicapped. It is important to distinguish the roles and duties of the home helps from the community care workers. The community care workers offer emotional and social support with some personal care, while the home helps do mostly household assistance, to which they add some emotional support and personal care. Obviously, there is some overlap between the two, but each reports to a different supervisor.

Referrals and Assessments

Referrals for community care can come from any source, although most come from physicians and hospitals. The home help organizer may also refer to community care if his or her assessment determines that additional assistance is needed. Upon referral, the community care organizer visits the client and applies a standardized assessment form to evaluate the client's medical, social, and mental abilities as well as the availability of informal support systems. Family members are usually present during this initial assessment. Reassessments are made every three months, but they can be more frequent if the condition warrants it.

Eligibility and Coverage

The goal of the program is to maintain the elderly in the community as long as possible; persons are referred to institutional care only if they constitute a danger to themselves or others. The only eligibility requirements are that the prospective client (1) would be eligible for admission to a long-stay hospital or old person's home, (2) is of retirement age, and (3) can initially be maintained at home (at a rate not to exceed £70 a week, in 1988). For terminal care, more expensive cases are often accepted.

Care is available twenty-four hours a day, seven days a week. If necessary, the organizer can purchase services that cannot be provided through the program, such as night care. Since the home helps work only until 11 P.M., overnight care must be separately budgeted.

Contributions by Clients

Clients are required to pay for the program and are assessed according to their incomes. The minimum contribution is £3.50 ($6.30) a week. Persons receiving a minimum attendance allowance must pay £4 (2.54) a week, and persons receiving the maximum allowance can pay up to £21 a week. The organizer makes the final decision regarding the payment.

Staffing

The community care workers who provide the direct service are supervised by organizers, mostly by telephone and occasional home visits. In 1988, there were 172 part-time workers, mostly middle-aged women, in the program. They are introduced individually to the clients by the organizer, who attempts to match worker to client. The workers usually have three cases per week, with individual contracts for each. The community care workers are paid £2.50 ($4.50) per visit Monday through Friday and £3.50 per visit on weekends and holidays and do not receive any benefits. Their turnover rate of 30 to 40 percent annually is rather high and stems from the unsteady nature of the work. Workers usually want clients in a specific geographic area, close to where they live. If a client dies or moves, and there is no other client immediately available, the worker does not get a new assignment. Because of this insecurity, many workers eventually leave for full-time employment in other fields. The workers are also encouraged to attend formal staff meetings. However, as these are not paid meetings, it is not feasible to make such attendance compulsory. Because of this, the organizers try to be very careful in their recruitment. Mature women, experienced in care-giving, are preferred.

LIVERPOOL

The city of Liverpool in the north of England provides another example of the organization and role of the home help service. Liverpool's decentralized home help program is divided into nine districts, with twenty-three organizers and 1,449 home helps located in each district. The organizers are responsible for the home helps and the administration of the program in their specific geographic areas. They, in turn, are supervised by a principal organizer, located in the central office of social services. This decentralized model facilitates the local organizer's accessibility to clients as well as the recruitment of home helps.

The organizer plays the role of primary case manager for the client, developing for each a unique plan. For each client there is a record card that specifies the services being used and the frequency of use.

Liverpool emphasizes home care as the preferable means of assistance for all persons. In fact, very few home care clients ever enter an institution. The program is ready, in fact, to extend as much care as required to maintain the client in the community.

Duties of the Home Help

In contrast to Dartford, home helps in Liverpool provide both domestic and personal assistance seven days a week, from 8 A.M. to 8 P.M., with special assistance available until 11 P.M. Tasks include meal preparation, fire lighting, bed making, shopping, and cleaning as well as bathing and dressing. The home helps are not permitted to administer medications, but they can supervise the client in taking them. If homes require intensive cleaning beyond the routine jobs, special cleaning teams are available. Presently, due to budget limitations, there are waiting lists for persons who are not identified as urgent cases or at risk of being institutionalized.

Referrals and Assessments

Referral for home help can be made by anyone, although most referrals come from physicians, hospitals, and family. Within twenty-four hours of a referral, the local organizer visits and makes the initial assessment as well as appropriate referrals to other agencies. The assessment evaluates the tasks that the client and family can do and what formal assistance is required.

There is no standard for determining the number of hours of home help for a client. The organizer decides independently, basing the decision upon specific client needs. The number of hours can range from two to fourteen per week, and may even be as high as thirty hours for specific cases. Reassessments are made every three months if the person is receiving daily home help and every six months if the assistance is less frequent.

Funding and Staffing

The home help service receives a budget of £5,000,000 ($9,000,000) per year and services approximately 5,000 clients a day. The average cost per client is £20 ($36.00) per week (1988), which makes the service considerably less expensive than the average nursing home, at a cost of £187 ($336.00) per week. Services, provided free to the clients, are paid for out of local taxes and grants. If the client does receive the government's attendance allowance, this money, unlike in the Kent program, is not appropriated by the home help service.

The home help workers are paid by the hour and usually work 19.5 hours a week at the rate of £2.50 an hour ($4.50), visiting four to five clients a day. They are unionized government employees and receive the standard benefits and pensions.

There are no educational requirements for home helps, but the service prefers persons who have had experience as care givers. As found in most areas, the majority are women in their midforties with grown children. Because of the high unemployment rate in the region, there is little difficulty in either recruiting or retaining home helps.

Training

Liverpool has begun to emphasize the importance of training for home care workers. The home helps receive an initial induction course of two hours and spend one week working with an experienced home help. Many also take a basic college course in family care, which is offered four hours a day for twelve weeks. Persons who take an advanced course can receive a diploma after twelve months of study. Every three months all home helps receive a two-week in-service training, which is given by the department of social services.

Coordination with Hospitals

A particularly innovative part of the Liverpool program is its Home from Hospitals initiative, begun in 1974 to assist hospitalized elderly persons when returning home.

Patients who will need care at discharge are directly referred to one of the project's organizers by the hospital social workers. The organizer assesses the patient while in the hospital and visits the home before the discharge. Once back home, the patient is eligible to receive up to four weeks of four-hour daily intensive care. At the end of that period, the district home help organizer determines whether the person requires continued service. This program has greatly improved the integration of the hospital with community services to provide immediate care for the elderly during a vulnerable period.

BEXLEY COMMUNITY CARE SCHEME

The Bexley Community Care Scheme was started in June 1984 to provide services not offered through the usual statutory social services and health departments by improving and strengthening the natural informal caring network of frail elderly. Rather than providing direct services, the scheme seeks to activate and organize community persons to perform helping tasks. The role of the case manager is to assist the client and family to locate both resources and community helpers. Upon receiving a request for services, the scheme's community care manager makes a home visit and assesses the needs of the client, usually in conjunction with the family.

A significant feature of the scheme is that whenever possible, the client or the principal care giver takes on the hiring of the attendant. Most of the funding comes from grants or from the attendance allowance received by each client. The scheme also trains the families to identify governmental benefits for which they might be eligible and which can be applied to pay for the costs of assistance.

The overall goal is to have the families become the case managers, with the coordinator only assisting them in developing the care plans. Once this care plan is written, a copy goes to the family or client. The coordinator plays a minimal role in monitoring the plan. If necessary, case meetings can be held weekly, but most cases are monitored once every three months. If there are no problems, this monitoring may be even done by telephone.

This scheme is unique in that the agency plays a secondary role in the implementation of the services. It builds instead on the skills and abilities of the informal network. It seeks to demonstrate that through careful education and guidance, families can effectively help and maintain bonds with their frail relatives.

The success of the scheme and its ability to save the local authority funds for domiciliary care have led to its expansion. Two new case managers were recruited in 1988, and the caseload was increased to sixty clients.

THE LIVERPOOL INTENSIVE DOMICILIARY
CARE SCHEME

The Liverpool Intensive Domiciliary Care Scheme for Elderly Mentally Ill People was established in June 1981 by Age Concern of England. It was financed with assistance from the Liverpool City Council and the Liverpool Health Authority. Funding for the scheme was renewed in 1988 for an additional seven years. The scheme provides comprehensive community care to twenty-five dementia victims, who are assisted by fifty-one trained aides under the direction of a coordinator. The beneficiaries are not required to pay for the services.

In most cases two to three aides work with each client on a rotation basis to ensure both continuity of care and respite for the workers. Due to the needs of dementia sufferers, it is important that they receive consistent care from the same workers. Too many workers rotating in the home could aggravate the patient's confusion. There is no time limit to the services, and some clients have been in the scheme for several years. Each client receives five hours of care a day, between 8 A.M. and 10 P.M., seven days a week. The usual pattern consists of a long visit in the morning and a shorter one in the late afternoon or evening.

There is on the average a three-month waiting list for care, although those at risk of being institutionalized are accepted immediately. Care late at night is a possibility only if deemed essential.

Referrals and Assessment

Referrals to the service may come from anyone, but they are usually initiated by a physician. Upon referral, the psychiatric nurse and the program coordinator make an assessment of the client at home. There is no standardized form, but potential beneficiaries are judged as to whether they can be motivated or helped by this intense service. The main objective is to induce them to function somewhat independently.

If the person is determined eligible for care, he or she is referred to a psychogeriatrician for further evaluation. Reassessments are made every six months.

Training and Salaries

The aides receive a two-week training course in mental health. The majority of the aides are mature women, many of whom have worked in nursing homes. Once accepted into the program, they work with experienced aides for two weeks before receiving their own cases. As with the home helps, there is no recruitment problem in the Liverpool area.

The pay rate, £2.90 ($5.22) an hour, surpasses that of workers in residential care or nursing homes. The aides also receive extra pay for nights and weekends and double pay for Sundays. The average work week is 17.5 hours. Clients are matched as much as possible with the workers.

Supervision

Unlike standard home help programs, the scheme is built on close monitoring and supervision. The director visits each client at home once a week. Small group meetings of the home helpers are held monthly for further supervision and training. All of the workers can reach the director at home by phone, whenever needed. This informality, flexibility, and close contact are regarded as essential to the program's effectiveness.

The actual costs of the program are comparable to those of care in a nursing home. It is estimated that one case costs approximately £325 ($585.00) for four weeks, which is about £4 less than a bed in a nursing home. However, according to the director, the standard of care that the person receives at home on a one-to-one basis surpasses the care in an institution. To date, the scheme has been found to successfully delay institutional care (University of Liverpool, 1986).

ACCESS: HOME SUPPORT FOR DEMENTIA SUFFERERS

Unlike the Liverpool scheme, which provides direct service, Access is a program providing only information, advice, and support for caregivers of dementia sufferers in the Ipswich area. As with the scheme in Liverpool, it also originated through joint funding from the local social services and health department, with additional funds from Age Concern and private grants. This joint support reflects the underlying premise that dementia sufferers are at the boundary between social services and health care, needing particular personal and domestic care to remain in the community.

Many of these patients live alone, without family care givers. Moreover, in those instances where care givers are present, they are often found to be very old themselves, with difficulties in coping with the patient's disability.

The program consequently helps both the elderly and their care givers through a case management approach that develops liaisons with appropriate community services. Presently, it is staffed by a coordinator, a social worker, a community psychiatric nurse, and a secretary. Each of the professionals may assume the case management task for a given client.

Most of the requests for services are initiated by families and are reviewed on a weekly basis. The professional that conducts the home visit becomes the case manager and sets up the care plan, which may consist of day care, home help, respite care, psychiatric care, or psychiatric assessment, depending on the availability of a functioning care giver.

As of 1988 the project carried 150 cases, with the nurse and social worker responsible for approximately 65 each and the director overseeing the balance of 20. The social worker and the nurse perform similar, in-distinguishable forms of case management, but given that the psychiatric nurse is paid by the health department while the social worker's salary is covered by the social services department, some problems with bound-aries occasionally surface at the administrative level. At the program level, the two workers collaborate closely.

Because Access does not provide direct services, it must depend on the district nurses and home helps. Yet, the number of hours of care per week allocated to Access clients may or may not coincide with the assessed need initially made by the Access staff. To supplement their assistance, the program initiates its own fund-raising to provide a budget for extra help such as putting a client to bed. This assistance can facilitate main-taining a person in the community, but it is not covered by the local authority. The Access staff often intervenes and finds a neighbor or other person who will take on this nightly duty.

The evaluation of the original research project indicated that with sup-port many dementia sufferers can be kept in their natural communities (Askham et al., 1987). In almost all cases, Access was able to attend to these persons at a weekly cost significantly lower than that of a psychiatric hospital or residential care home.

VOLUNTARY AGENCIES

In addition to statutory or governmental initiatives, there are also innovative programs supported by voluntary agencies. One of the largest and most extensive is Crossroads, which provides care attendants to handicapped persons living in the community on a nationwide basis. Al-though age is not a criterion for eligibility, over 75 percent of the clients are elderly.

Crossroads seeks to prevent institutionalization by helping families to reduce the risk of their breakdown. It also aims to supplement existing statutory services and to enhance high standards of community care.

Much of the assistance is provided to elderly frail persons at risk of being institutionalized because they did not qualify for the statutory ser-vices. These are persons who, because they have a care giver in the home, may not, in some areas, receive traditional home care. Moreover, in many instances these care givers are themselves elderly and frail, and thus are not able to provide the needed assistance. Crossroads fills in the gap in service provision, on a 24-hour-a-day basis.

The program consists of 133 schemes organized in eight local regions throughout the country. Each scheme is autonomous and is administered by a coordinator. It pays an affiliation fee to the national association and receives local funds through joint financing from the Department of Health and social security.

In setting up a local scheme, a proposal or application for funds is made to the local health or social services departments by a committee of local representatives. The specific plans are based on demographic and need indicators in the local areas. A Crossroads scheme will not be established if its services are duplicating an existing program.

The coordinators recruit six to ten care attendants, whose main qualifying requirement is that they have had some experience in caring for others usually through nursing or working with the disabled. In establishing a new scheme, the regional director may be involved with the coordinator in the initial hiring. The attendants are required to be ready for a full twenty-four hour day, if needed in special circumstances.

Attendants are assigned to relieve the primary care giver and offer substitute care, including both nursing and personal care. The bulk of the attendant's tasks consists of bathing, toileting, incontinence care, and feeding. Furthermore, the attendant may provide only respite care while the caregiver is out of the home.

Attendants are paid by the hour and their wages are comparable to those of home care workers in the local services, but they do not get benefits. Each client receives an average of six to eight care hours a week.

All attendants are trained in handling, lifting, health, and safety as well as special conditions diagnosed in their impending caseload. Once they have completed the training, the attendants tend to stay with the program, resulting in a low turnover rate.

The coordinators conduct monthly visits to evaluate and reassess the patient's conditions. During these visits families may communicate their own evaluations of the workers' performance, but they are often reluctant to complain because they fear losing the help they receive.

Funding

Clients are not required to pay for Crossroads services, although some make nominal contributions of £1 to £2 pounds per visit. Coordinators can decide to charge, but as it is difficult to assess financial status, the services are usually provided free.

The average cost of a visit or unit of service is approximately £5 ($9.00) an hour, which is comparable to that of the statutory services. Some schemes do private fund-raising and also seek funds from the local health and social services departments.

OTHER MODELS OF HOME CARE

New models of home care services, such as the STAT (Supplemental Home Care Foundation) in the Netherlands, are being spearheaded and partially supported by the National Cross Association as well as by the Family Care Association and private insurance companies, who see it as an alternate or substitute for the more costly institutional care. Its patients require more complex care than is normally provided at home.

The STAT has been in existence since November 1987, and is currently operating in only seven districts of the county. It provides a maximum of three months of twenty-four hour care for terminal cases or for rehabilitation after hospitalization. Long-term chronic care cases are excluded.

The referral is made to a local nurse, who subsequently conducts a home assessment. This evaluation differs from that of the National Cross Association: it investigates more closely what the family and neighbors are able to do for the patient, while the Cross assessment looks primarily at what the patient needs. The STAT form also aims to determine whether there is a family member who can be responsible for coordinating the patient's care.

Most of the STAT personnel are women who want to work only part-time. They have had some paraprofessional training but are not required to be nurses. Because the program is concentrated in the regions with high unemployment rates, there has been little problem with recruitment. The program also includes an extensive network of volunteers. The STAT workers, who are available twenty-four hours a day, are required to keep logbooks that remain in the client's house. The books list the tasks completed and any changes or problems in the client's condition.

Family care, another experiment, is jointly sponsored by the provincial Cross Association and the Home Help Association of Hellewag. It provides extra care to persons who are at risk of being institutionalized and whose needs exceed the services the Cross can ordinarily provide. Teams of two or three home helps are assigned to clusters of approximately ten elderly living near each other. The team coordinates tasks and fills in the gaps in care that might commonly exist. District supervisors draw the care plans and reassess them periodically, according to the complexity of each case.

ALMERE

Almere is a new town created in the early 1980s. It is approximately 30 miles from Amsterdam and has a population of 57,300. Because of its newness, the government has been interested in experimenting with a new system of services. The Project Health Care Almere was initiated in 1983 under the auspices of the Ministry of Welfare, Health, and Cultural Affairs and the Almere Council. Its aim was to create a coordinated system of health services centered around a primary health care team. Funding was provided by the central government and the private health insurance associations.

As of January 1988, all of the primary health providers—nurses, physicians, social workers, physiotherapists, and home helps—have been placed under a single authority called Primary Care Benefits of Almere (Eerstelijns Voorzieningen Almere [EVA]). All of these personnel except the home helps are distributed in eleven health centers.

Home Helps

The home help system under EVA operates through three districts with three to four supervisors in each district. Each oversees approximately fifty home helps. These supervisors rotate in assuming the role of manager for the district. The manager makes the initial assessments and develops the care plan for each client. Coordination is basic to the system. The group of supervisors frequently discuss their cases with each other and are available to meet daily with the home helps. Formal meetings with the home helps take place every three weeks. Weekly conferences with the central home help administrator are held to discuss plans and issues.

Reassessments take place according to the intensity of care. For services that exceed twenty hours a week, reassessments are made weekly; if care is required eight to twenty hours a week, the reevaluation is made every three months, and if it consists of less than eight hours a week, the interval between reevaluations may be extended to six months.

A home help visits approximately three to five cases a week. However, some of these persons are seen as often as three times a day; thus a home help can easily work forty to fifty hours a week. The usual hours of work are 8 A.M. to 10 P.M., although occasional overnight care is possible.

Home nursing is provided through the National Cross Association, although in Almere the director is a part of the administrative structure of EVA. The Cross nurses are dispersed in the eleven health centers. As in other parts of the country, referrals for home nursing are usually made by a physician. The district nurse in the local center makes the standard assessment of needs and develops the care plan accordingly. Often the nurse making the plan is the person who provides the care. Visits must not exceed a maximum of three times a day, and reassessments must be made at least every three months.

Although both the home helps and the nurses work for EVA, it is not always clear which professional discipline takes on the role of case manager. Presently, decisions tend to be made informally on a case-by-case basis. Because conflicts may arise, plans are being made to standardize these relationships and specify criteria for determining client responsibility. The association is developing one assessment form that will be used by both the nurses and the home helps, and is expected to facilitate cooperation.

The distinguishing strength of the EVA program is that it has broken down the formal barriers between the National Cross Association and the Home Help Association. With both now operating under a single administrative structure, coordination of tasks can in principle be systematized. Financing procedures, however, continue to undermine these coordinative efforts. The salary of the home helps remains much lower than that of the nurses. This disparity perpetuates their lower status while it also limits the volume and types of services they are authorized to provide.

OTHER EXPERIMENTS IN HOME CARE

As a part of the governmental policy shift from institutional to community care, five research and experimental service projects are being initiated in different parts of the Netherlands. They will be closely monitored, and the successful ones will be replicated throughout the country. Following are brief descriptions of these projects.

In Rotterdam, a project initiated in May 1988 is comparing the wellbeing and mortality rates of older persons in homes for the aged with those in the community. The study is using an experimental design in which seventy-five persons making applications to institutions will be cared for at home with extensive services under the supervision of a case manager. These persons will be compared with a matched control group of patients admitted to an institution as well as a control group of patients who are neither admitted or receiving extra home care. Measurements of the wellbeing status, morbidity, and mortality rates of the three groups will be made at three different intervals.

A project in Nieuwegein is investigating the advantage of having one screening instrument and one local board make the assessment for either home care or nursing home care. Two groups of persons will be followed, those admitted to a home and those receiving home care services. Two observations will be made of these groups, one at the time of application and one two months after admission to a home or after home care has started. The evaluation will make structured comparison between the groups to determine whether careful and comprehensive screening and assessment can reduce the rates of institutionalization.

Given that coordination between services remains a problem throughout the country, a project in Groningen will implement a new method of cooperation between the home helps, nurses, and local general practitioners. The current status of the coordination of these services is being evaluated. Based upon the findings of the evaluation, a new model for coordination will be designed and implemented.

A project in Bevelanden is attempting to evaluate the effectiveness of substituting day care for institutional care. Two nursing homes and six homes for the aged are being remodeled to have fewer beds, with space being provided for day care. The objective is to show that day care can be less costly than institutional care, yet just as effective.

The Ouderenbelied Venlo project is focusing on the involvement of elderly persons as advocates and spokesmen at local community boards. These are forums that review services and propose new types of specific services they feel are needed. The boards will also make recommendations regarding the organization of these services. Moreover, they will be involved in reviewing applications of persons to homes for the aged, indicating how they feel such applications should be prioritized.

HOSPITAL PRIVADO DE LA COMUNIDAD

The central role of the physicians in Argentina's home care system has also been extended to provide "home hospitalization." Located in Mar del Plata, a city of 500,000 inhabitants 250 miles south of Buenos Aires, the Hospital Privado de la Comunidad is a nonprofit medical facility owned and sponsored by the community. It has contractual agreements for the provision of secondary (hospitalization) services with the governmental Institute of Social Services, and it also acts as an HMO for almost seventy thousand affiliated persons.

The hospital has adapted the "home hospitalization" concept previously designed by the Italian Hospital of the city of Buenos Aires. It fosters very early discharges, even after complex surgical procedures. The hospital relies for this on (1) a highly mobile and flexible team of nurses and nurse practitioners, (2) the active involvement of a "trainable" family, and (3) a special unit of home-visiting physicians who provide the linkage, during the home convalescence stage, between the primary-care physician and the hospital's attending medical team. This bridging function is facilitated by the fact that the hospital operates at both the primary and secondary levels of care. Patients' primary-care physicians are full-time hospital staff members. This is a health maintenance organization model of service, the only difference being that elderly patients do not pay on a private basis. The hospital is reimbursed instead by the federal government's insurance program, PAMI.

Because the hospital is aware that primary-care physicians do not have the time for thorough follow-ups in the patients' homes, it established a special department of full-time, home-visiting physicians. Part of their duties is to alert the primary physician and the attending ones at the hospital about each patient's progress. They treat the patient in their homes and also act as the convenors of multidisciplinary teams of medical specialists, physical and occupational therapists, social workers, and homemakers, who also visit the patients in their homes.

Home care operates as a freestanding service within the hospital's nursing department. It coordinates all the above-mentioned medical resources, that is, the primary, secondary and home-visiting physicians; nurses; physical and occupational therapists; paramedical social services; and the ancillary home attendants.

Direct referrals for home care are evaluated by a team consisting of a physician, an attending nurse, and a hospital social worker. Their recommendations require final approval from the hospital's administration, a procedure that may appear to be an infringement of the team's professional discretion or expertise. It is, however, a fiscal step that responds to eligibility considerations. The administration determines whether the hospital will assume the costs, in the case of lack of coverage, or whether it will route the case to other more pertinent programs in the community.

The hospital-based primary-care physician subsequently decides on the termination of home care services. This may come about when the patient's condition has improved or, conversely, when institutional care is imperative. A major determinant of the latter is when both the primary-care physician and the social worker verify that the family is no longer a viable support system or that it refuses to continue assisting the relative and/or refuses to cooperate with the home care team.

Are these innovative initiatives meeting their intended objectives? The same question may be posed in the case of the regular, ongoing programs. The extent to which they are properly evaluated and satisfy their clients' needs is examined in the next chapter.

8

Evaluation, Quality of Care, and Advocacy

How effective are the home care programs in the countries under study? While the question is frequently raised in service-related quarters, systematic evaluations are not generalized occurrences and are seldom required as a condition for funding. The main thrust has been in launching home care and providing services, but some resources have been allocated for assessing their results.

Evaluations are a low priority because it is generally assumed that home-delivered services are less expensive than institutional care and that they respond much better to the clients' preference to remain at home. Regardless of whether the choice between institutional and home care is made on philosophical or cost-effectiveness grounds, all countries uphold the criterion that keeping the old or disabled client at home is the most desirable outcome.

Specialized services that are linked to teaching hospitals or academic institutions or which have been initiated as special demonstrations tend, almost as a rule, to incorporate evaluative requirements. On the other hand, services mandated by law and lodged in the public sector have little incentive to assess on a regular basis whether they are meeting their objectives. As private-sector providers begin making inroads, often under service contracts, the pressure to institute quality-of-care norms, licensing regulations, and cost-effectiveness measures is mounting. This chapter reflects the incipient and still very uneven developments in program evaluation and quality-of-care standards. It also incorporates the sporadic manifestations of policy analysis and advocacy initiated at the grass-roots level by consumer groups.

NORWAY

Home care in Norway must be understood and evaluated in terms of the country's system of government, which leaves to the discretion of each municipality the design of its own system of social services within a broad national legislative framework. There is not, therefore, a single or universal model of home care services. Given that there are 453 local governments, it is conceivable that hundreds of such service models could have evolved. This, however, has not been the case. Some municipalities do engage in original experimentation, but most borrow from each other's experience. As a result, the degree of variation in the resulting models of home care services is rather limited.

The policy of decentralization recently initiated requires that municipalities further distribute their services in smaller and autonomous geographical units, or district offices. This administrative approach entails a more flexible coordination between local agencies, professionals, and auxiliary personnel. It assumes that service workers will operate in multidisciplinary teams and that elderly clients will have easier access to a wide range of services emanating from a single one-stop service center. Moreover, it expects that district staff will be able to act immediately, without having either to negotiate professional boundaries or to ascertain complex eligibility requirements. The decision making is thus delegated to the district office without need for confirmation or authorization from above. Determining the extent to which this rather high order of expectations is accomplished will require carefully designed evaluations. The city of Oslo has already experimented for three years in four of its projected twenty-five districts. The evaluation revealed that problems of outreach and accessibility remained difficult to overcome, as isolated and low-income persons who never used services still did not avail themselves of much-needed formal supports. The more educated and economically better off, however, maximized the use of public services.

Home help is by far the largest service offered to the aged in Norway, as it covers about 70 percent of all home care. Home nursing, though, is the fastest-growing service, due to the fact that admission rates to institutional care are being slightly but deliberately reduced.

Home care has been historically shaped by a medical or nursing model, and nurses still perform its leading roles. With decentralization, a social dimension has been added. Its intent is to address the total needs of the client population, not just particular illnesses. Moreover, patients are given a chance to participate in decisions concerning their treatment.

Norway has a tradition of paid provision of home care by relatives. Current policy, while attentive to the need for a more predictable, larger-scale, professionalized service system, does not want to do away with family care givers. On the contrary, it seeks to offer them financial incentives so they remain an organic component of the service system. The central government expects that this strategy will both reduce costs and alleviate the present shortage of home care workers.

Some municipalities are also experimenting with a different set of manpower strategies aimed at recruiting a more stable home care work force. Paid training of up to one year, correspondence courses, paid travel time, and full fringe benefits for part-time workers are only a few examples. It is not clear yet whether all these manpower strategies will succeed. Recruitment of spouses of foreign workers are additional approaches that recently have been debated.

Home care and community-based services are being given more weight than institutional care. Nursing homes will not be entirely phased out, but their very mission is being substantially altered. They are to become the seat for flexible service pools adapted for the provision of home care and short-term rehabilitation or treatment of the home care recipient. The home nurse often provides continuity of care by attending to patients both at home and during their short stays in the nursing home.

It must be borne in mind too, that home care and institutional care are not always conceived as antithetical terms, but rather as two interchangeable or complementary services linked by the assignment of the same workers to both. Many municipalities resort to the "open care" approach, whereby patients alternate between the two services according to need and are followed by the same staff. The nursing home contracts and expands in both bed occupancy and staffing patterns depending on how many home care patients are being transitorily placed for short-term rehabilitation or intensive therapy. There is no concern about filling beds. Patients keep rotating from home to nursing home, but for the most part it is anticipated that they will return to their own homes. Moreover, families are prepared at the time of admission for the forthcoming discharge and the subsequent provision of home care services. If needed, the municipality assists, to ensure that patients retain their homes and can return to them.

In essence, Norway's nursing-oriented model of home care incorporates a more fluid, even interchangeable, pattern of multidisciplinary team work. Instead of the sequential long-term care continuum prevalent in the United States, whereby patients escalate progressively from services for the moderately frail to those for the totally dependent, some Norwegian municipalities are experimenting with a rather syncretic model that revolves around each individual's needs. They no longer separately employ home care workers and nursing home personnel, or for that matter senior-center personnel; instead, all personnel share in the same enterprise. This system cannot be improvised easily. It requires relentless planning, continuous training, mutual trust among service professionals, and, especially, total commitment. This approach is also costly, at least in the short run. Both central government and municipal officials expect, however, that costs will in the long run be reduced, once the need for indefinite institutionalization is curtailed. Norway is involved in a very original and far-reaching experiment. The extent to which it succeeds, as well as the lessons to be learned from it, await a comprehensive evaluation.

SWEDEN

Home care is also the fastest-growing service for the aged in Sweden, but there is no unanimous approval of the way it was designed and how it operates. Policy analysts, service providers, and evaluators have observed that it is overorganized, that it tries unrealistically to satisfy too many clients' needs, and that in the process it thwarts the workers' sense of initiative and their capacity for decision making.

It has also been expressed that it rests on an idyllic vision of the aging process. The assumption that most if not all older persons can be kept active and alert through open and community care is not borne out by the demographic indicators that point to an increasingly older and sicker population. Moreover, home care is occupationally redefined in a way that does not respond to the clients' most stringent needs. In an attempt to upgrade the status of home care workers as well as to make their position more attractive to younger persons, new workers are trained to underplay cleaning and scrubbing and to provide instead more socialization and companionship. This, however, is not what the consumers expect to receive.

Part of the problem stems from a deliberate strategy aimed at convincing a new cadre of younger workers that home care can offer them a promising career. Critics feel, however, that these efforts have little chance of success. To begin with, home care is the occupational choice of last resort for most young persons in a highly industrialized country that is already experiencing severe personnel shortages in better-paying fields.

Second, young home care workers seem to have great difficulty in handling senile dementia, multiple chronicity, and the sheer physical pressures of the job all at once. Furthermore, a home helper usually works alone and never knows what to expect when arriving at a client's home.

Finding a person who is acting out, slumped in a chair in a state of deep depression, or even worse, lying on the floor unconscious, could be too much for an eighteen-year-old to handle. It is not surprising, therefore, that young workers quit in droves, despite all incentives and supports.

Finally, elderly clients may, in turn, find it difficult to socialize with persons who are younger than their own grandchildren. They are specially reluctant to undress in front of these young workers and let them give baths or change diapers.

Eliasson (1988) found that home helpers in Stockholm establish better continuity of care and personal ties with clients residing at home than with those in the service houses. The worker assumes, in the first instance, more of a professional and therapeutic concern toward the frail person, and wishes to alter any adverse circumstances. It is different in service houses because the teams tend to gravitate toward an institutionalized model and operate in a conveyor-belt fashion. Their schedules may be more efficient, but the client is no longer treated in a holistic way.

Depersonalization is the inevitable corollary when team members divide among themselves the tasks in more specialized components. Eliasson writes about the "mutual burning out" of clients and workers when the possibility of getting to know each other as people is not attainable. Szebehely (1988) attributes workers' discouragement and burnout to the fact that they seldom manage to complete a job. They feel that they rush in and rush out, treating their clients as marginal beings, that they have no time to relate to clients' personal concerns. It is not a matter of training but of time allocation and work organization. The more extensive and systematic the training home helpers receive, the higher the chances they will drop out. The better-trained ones perceive more readily the discrepancy between what ought to be done and that which is possible in the minimal allotted time. Szebehely considers it also wrong to assume that all home helpers need or wish to upgrade their professional status.

It is also unwise to advocate workers adopt a "therapeutic" model of intervention. The chances that they will succeed in changing the personality makeup of a ninety-year-old man and get him to start cleaning his home when he never did before are rather remote. What workers need, according to Szebehely, is a more focused but smaller caseload and continuity of contact with the same clients rather than the sporadic contact produced by the present rotational schedules.

Several proposals have been made to change the planning course of home care, including the following:

1. Abandon the "young workers" strategy and revert to the old-fashioned practice of the sixties and seventies of paying relatives. Only 7 percent of home care was delivered by paid family mem-

bers in 1986, as contrasted with 25 percent in 1970. This resulted from the central government's systematic policy of professionalizing home care and staffing it with full-time workers.

2. Send in home care workers in teams of two, so that both the socialization and household chores can be attended to simultaneously. Two home care workers instead of one may appear to be more expensive, but teamwork will enhance morale and ultimately reduce absenteeism, drop-out rates, and especially, recruitment and training costs.

3. Admit that institutional care may well be the most humane solution for many lonely and frail older persons. A nursing home will provide them round-the-clock attention, for 168 hours a week. When at home, they seldom receive more than 15 hours a week of home care services. It is obvious that in the absence of family or friends, they will be alone for the remaining 153 hours of the week. The policy objectives of "normalization," "integrity," and "self-determination" spelled out in the 1982 Social Services Act are of little relevance for many of these lonely and incapacitated persons. They would gladly trade their alleged normality for more security and continuity of care. There is little doubt, in the view of many analysts and service providers, that these goals can be better met in long-term care facilities.

4. Break up the home care job in three components as follows: (a) contract out the heavy household tasks to commercial home cleaning companies, (b) recruit part-time employees from middle-aged persons for the lighter chores, and (c) have social workers involve informal supports, namely family members, neighbors, friendly visitors, and so forth, in socialization, escorting, and companionship.

Whatever course is followed, it will have to come to grips with the political posturing of the last two decades. The parties of the left have argued that people who paid taxes all their lives should not have to depend on the charity and good will of volunteers and that it is the state's ultimate responsibility to both guarantee and deliver their benefits. Unions have also contributed to remove the families' paid helping roles with their demand for full-time employment and professionalization. The parties of the right, in contrast, want to bring in the private sector and give more discretion to individual consumers regarding how and where they wish to purchase the services they need. They suggest instituting both a voucher and a purchase-of-services system to this effect.

Government officials are particularly concerned that despite the tax-equalization grants aimed at reducing the disparities in resources between wealthier and poorer municipalities, the gap keeps widening. The decentralization philosophy and objectives underlying the country's framework laws have produced a host of unexpected inequities, which make a mockery of the principle that a person is entitled to the same level of welfare regardless of his or her place of residence. Furthermore, counties and municipalities are not working effectively together. Their level of cooperation and joint planning is sporadic, and on occasion nonexistent. Central-government officials are proposing making coordination legally mandatory and transferring old age care to local governments. As far as home care services are concerned, they anticipate the need for the following:

1. A closer link between housing renovation and development for the aged and disabled on one hand, and home care on the other. It makes no sense to "normalize" a person in his or her environment if the quality of the latter is deficient or not conducive to normal and secure living. This is being currently tested in experiments like the previously mentioned one in Nörkoping. (See Chapter 6)

2. A greater emphasis on cost-effectiveness, without necessarily denying clients their basic rights to self-determination and normalization.

3. A transfer of resources from county councils to municipalities, in order to better meet needs for housing and home-delivered services.

4. More effective coordination between county councils and municipalities, and even the joint operation of the home help (municipal) and home health care (county) services under a unified municipal authority.

5. A change in the fiscal formulas for tax redistribution and central-government grants aimed at equalizing service resources across municipalities.

6. A gradual transition from service houses to smaller congregate units of about five to six older persons living in a regular apartment and receiving home services. The housing units geared for psychiatric and developmental disabled cases will be kept separate from those reserved for average older residents.

7. An intensification of training and professional upgrading of the present human resources in home care.

8. A greater attention to quality standards. Municipalities have been very concerned with ensuring that services are actually provided, but do not like to assess quality. They certainly have

no tradition or awareness of cost-effectiveness considerations. Rather than spreading services thinly to too many recipients, they will have to focus on fewer critical cases. A selective approach will have to be accompanied by systematic program evaluation in order to justify their more rigorous service priorities.

Advocacy in Sweden: The Stockholm Cooperative for Independent Living

STIL stands for Stockholm's Independent Living Group. It is an advocacy organization of handicapped people created in 1983 with the goal of expanding the range of personal-assistance alternatives available to persons with serious disabilities. Members demand, among other things, the right to do their own hiring of home care workers and to control the funds the municipality would normally allocate to this effect.

Legally constituted as a cooperative, STIL requested a purchase-of-services contract arrangement with the city. This would have meant that STIL would gain administrative control over the entire service delivery process affecting its members. The city viewed this request, along with the concepts of grass-roots advocacy and consumer control, as a substantial departure from established procedures. It reluctantly gave in, but it never conceded that it was awarding a purchase-of-services contract. It referred to it instead as an "experiment," diluted among several dozens of other service demonstrations.

STIL also had to overcome the resistance of organized labor, which has persistently been fighting for the professionalization of home care services. The latter entails a demand for more training, full-time employment, job security, more fringe benefits, and the prospects of a career ladder. Ratzka (1986) reported that the political left was particularly antagonistic because they viewed consumers' movements as highly individualistic and resented the notion of personal assistance being removed from the public domain and placed in the hands of private, or even profit-oriented, interests. Furthermore, STIL was labeled as an elitist movement. Its demand to have its members act as employers of their home care workers sounded as if they belonged to or identified with the upper economic strata of society.

For STIL the struggle was also conceived in class terms, but in its perception the handicapped were getting short shrift. STIL consequently sought to rectify the unbalanced distribution of power between service providers and consumers in favor of the latter. Moreover, members claimed that as consumers they knew what worked best for them and that furthering the professionalization of home care workers, as demanded by the unions and the local authorities, would aggravate the dependent status of the handicapped. They preferred instead a more flexible recruitment of part-time persons, particularly those looking for additional employment as a means to supplement other sources of income. Both the city and the unions opposed this approach, but they were careful to steer away from a head-on confrontation. They realized that it would not be good for their image to take on a small group of handicapped people.

The intended professionalization of home helpers, in STIL's view, would be bound to lead to a stifling bureaucratic regimentation and adherence to regulations over which consumers have little or no say. It would place all control in the public-service agencies and ultimately deprive consumers of the right to influence decisions affecting their own lives. In the best of circumstances, all consumers could do would be to lodge protests and appeals. Some partial improvements could be obtained, but service users would never succeed on the whole in rectifying the power imbalance. If somebody requires training, the STIL leadership added, it is not the workers but the consumers themselves. They should learn how to better assess what their needs are, and then how to select their best possible helpers. As for the latter, consumers want ordinary people like themselves, preferably their friends, relatives, or neighbors. They do not want to be patronized by do-gooders and samaritans.

Following the same train of thought, STIL has argued against the philosophy of case management. Members categorically refuse as individuals to become someone else's "case." Accepting this would be tantamount to subordination and admission of incompetence. They view themselves instead as employers and as producers of work opportunities. They wish, therefore, to plan their own schedules, negotiate with potential helpers, and decide how to use more efficiently the city's monetary allocation. STIL's trump card is that after four years of independent operation, they were able to demonstrate that they could set services in motion at a lower cost than the public sector, that they substantially reduced the city's administrative overhead costs, and that they could function as effective subcontractors.

No service system can be universal, STIL admits, and they realize that their model may not be applicable to all potential consumers, especially older persons. To begin with, they point to a de facto generational barrier. Elderly consumers for the most part seldom complain. Instead, they are thankful for whatever is handed to them. Also, there are too many senile dementia patients that do need to be managed and protected. STIL objects, however, that the city authorities perceive all handicapped people as similarly incompetent. The city, in their view, assumes that because a person is physically handicapped, he or she must also be mentally dependent. This attitude reduces all of the handicapped to the lowest possible denominator, as if they were all afflicted with advanced Alzheimer's disease.

STIL has resisted all attempts to be co-opted into the city's planning process, and has even refused to participate as a consumer's representative in municipal committees or forums. It has made instead the strategical decision to stay outside, as an independent watchdog. The group feels it can be more effective by relating to the city in an adversarial capacity. This has been hard for many municipal leaders to comprehend, particularly since there are few precedents and practically no tradition of consumer advocacy movements in Sweden.

City government officials have felt both troubled and ambivalent about STIL. One one hand, they recognize that it offers a positive alternative: it demonstrated that it can recruit its own home care workers and reduce costs by pooling the service needs of its members in a true cooperative fashion. And above all it relieved the city of all the related administrative chores. On the other hand, STIL remains a source of irritation because it has politicized the service-delivery process. The city authorities particularly resent its confrontational tactics and its unwillingness to compromise amicably at the negotiating table. When STIL does not get what it wants, all it has to do is threaten to repeat its first successful public demonstration. It then brought all members downtown in their wheelchairs to block traffic and effectively paralyzed Stockholm's business center, creating a scene that shocked city residents and received front-page coverage. The municipal authorities would not like to have the scene repeated. STIL is very aware of its bargaining power, and knows how to use it.

ENGLAND

England's governmental involvement in the implementation of home help services consists for the most part in awarding grants, setting guidelines, and collecting information on the quantity and scope (rather than on the quality) of services. Following their service-related statistics in depth, the government completes additional studies. Recommendations for services are also made, but local governments do not have to adopt them.

The 1986 study of the policy, resources, and management of the home help service (Department of Health and Social Security, 1987) is one example of such discrete evaluative undertaking. It examined home help services in eight county social service departments, looking primarily at their effectiveness, efficiency, and contribution to community care. The eight selected counties were all involved in developing flexible and intensive personal community care for persons who might otherwise be institutionalized. However, policy directions and strategies varied among the eight departments. The general pattern consisted of spreading services thinner, that is, offering fewer hours of service to more people. Clients received an average of 3.1 hours of home help service per week, with greater emphasis placed on domestic work than on personal or social care.

The study also found that the home help organizers in their role as case managers acted idiosyncratically, not according to any formal rules or standards. To begin with, the large caseloads, with an average of 210 per organizer, made the very task of case management nearly impossible. Also, there was little coordination between social workers, occupational therapists, and health professionals in developing individual care plans. Although good informal relationships between individual workers did evolve, no attempt was made to institute systematic collaborative procedures.

The study also noted the issue of training of home help organizers. In 1986 only 18.5 percent of home help organizers had appropriate professional qualifications. This lack of training was seen as a particular obstacle to effective service delivery, given that the complexity of clients' problems demanded commensurately sophisticated skills.

A final conclusion of the report was that the home help organizers were overloaded with too many duties. It called for more explicit guidelines as to the division of labor between case management, personnel work, budgeting, and administration. Moreover, it recommended that the county organizers be more involved in the formulation of local policies and the planning of services.

Evaluations are not a universal requirement for all home care programs. The extent to which they are designed and implemented depends on the initiatives adopted by local authorities, often in conjunction with a university research center. Innovative programs sponsored by private foundations or voluntary organizations may also initiate evaluation as part of their service demonstration. A case in point is the Access program, which extends information, advice, and support for care givers of dementia sufferers in the Ipswich area. As with the scheme in Liverpool, it also originated through joint funding from the local social services and health department, with additional contributions from Age Concern and private grants. This joint support reflected the project's underlying premise that dementia sufferers are at the boundary between social services and health care.

Access began as an action and research program in 1986 with the aim of developing the most effective means of maintaining persons who require both personal and domestic care in the community. Increasing numbers of dementia sufferers were living alone without family care givers. Moreover, care givers themselves were often elderly and found it increasingly difficult to cope with the patients.

During its research stage (1984–86), the program administered its own budget and could then recruit and train its own teams of home care workers. These workers overlapped in many ways with the traditional home helps, although they were given extra training in the management of dementia clients. The main difference from the regular home helps consisted in the scheduling flexibility of the Access home care workers, because they were available at all hours and stayed with the same clients. They could establish close and continuous relationships with them, often acting as surrogate family members. In addition to practical tasks, the workers also gave close emotional support to the clients and helped orient them to time and place as well as increase their social contacts.

A major change in the program occurred in 1986 with regard to its funding. Access no longer controls its own budget; instead, the funds are allocated by social services and all requests for assistance must go to the home help organizer employed by the social service department.

This has altered the original concept of the project, because Access no longer controls its own staff, and the home helps assigned by the Department of Social Services are not necessarily trained to work with this particular category of patients.

Evaluations tend to underscore the fear of loss of funding as the main concern, one that overwhelms many home care programs. There are no assurances that funds will remain constant or will increase to meet growing demand for services. Home care must compete with other social service programs for budgetary resources, and administrators must continuously document whether their programs adequately meet the needs of the elderly in their communities. At the same time, when encountering possible restraints, they must decide if and where to target their services. A secondary effect of the program change is the loss of morale among professional staff.

The central government's policy of encouraging private, for-profit agencies challenges the more traditional public sector, which has not yet been properly assessed. On the other hand, it is known that nonprofit agencies play a substantial role in augmenting the work of the government services. Crossroads, Access, and the National Association of Careers fill in the gaps in services not covered by the traditional programs. These groups are also able to act as advocates for clients and programs, pointing to emerging needs that are not being addressed by the public sector.

Home care programs in England are in a state of transition from the dominant public-sector organization to both private for-profit and voluntary organizations. If the central government chooses to relate to the local services through contractual mechanisms, quality-control regulations, and the encouragement of independent providers, home care as it has been traditionally known will become a matter of the past.

THE NETHERLANDS

Home care services are delivered by two national well-established agencies, the Central Home Help Association and the National Cross Association. The administrative structure of these organizations has proven to facilitate the experimentation with new modalities of service delivery and the adaptation of ongoing programs to fit local needs. The two agencies have thus fostered a considerable degree of flexibility and responsiveness, such as found in the "flying brigade" or hospital-discharge program in Amsterdam and the family care program in rural areas.

However, the perennial problem of coordination of those parallel organizations, as well as the overlap in the roles and duties of the home helps and the Cross nurses, remains unresolved. Despite these ongoing structural and operational problems, evaluative studies point to some outstanding innovative developments that merit consideration for transfer and replication. The method of hiring alpha helpers to provide domestic assistance reduces the costs of service, as these workers are hired directly by their clients rather than by the established agencies. Moreover, by working shorter hours and performing less skilled tasks, they free up the better-trained home helps to concentrate on more complex and demanding cases.

In 1988 the two national organizations were contemplating their eventual merger. The first order in their agenda was to achieve a more rational coordination and a concomitant reduction of blatant duplications. Quality-of-care and programs evaluation concerns were, however, less pressing. Although not totally absent, these concerns are currently attended to in a rather informal basis.

District managers monitor their teams of home help workers and, in most areas, design each patient's care plan and oversee its implementation. However, this supervisory function depends upon the manager's own expertise, since there are no written quality standards for home help care. Personal contacts and discussions with the home helps form the basis for evaluating the quality of the care. Moreover, there are no guidelines concerning the actual methodology and frequency of monitoring workers or for case assessment.

Administrative staff collect information on the number of persons served monthly, the total hours of work and persons employed, payments, hours of workers' leave, and the hours of training provided during the month. These data are submitted to and scrutinized by the Ministry of Welfare, Health and Culture, which is more concerned with the volume and extent of services provided than with their quality.

Individual client complaints about either the assessment or the care can be directed to either the team leader or the district manager. Clients have the right to request a new assessment or another worker. These complaints and the client's subsequent inputs constitute an additional component of the monitoring and evaluative process regarding the program and the individual home helps.

In the case of the home nursing service, each individual nurse prepares her own patient care plans, but nurses hold weekly team meetings to discuss and brainstorm about their cases and related problems. These meetings are supportive and consultative in nature, since the caseloads remain highly individualized.

No standardized quality-assessment methods of nursing care have so far been instituted. Monitoring of the individual nurses' work is done rather informally by their district managers. The nurses keep records on their individual cases and then transfer the information into monthly reports sent to the national association. Clients' complaints are first addressed to the nurse, but may then be appealed to the manager.

The National Cross Association has been particularly sensitive to quality-of-care and monitoring concerns and has sought to improve its procedures in these areas. One plan proposes assigning central-office inspectors to the districts to monitor the teams' quality of work. Another plan consists of having the team nurses supervise lower-level auxiliaries and generate with them standardized assessment forms. This plan would also assist in justifying the program's costs and substantiating eventual requests for more funds. As the Cross associations are beginning to experience the competition of small unlicensed agencies, the imperative to institute quality-of-care standards looms even greater.

There is no overall evaluation of the home help programs or their effectiveness in keeping persons at home. As stated earlier, the data collected is primarily focused on the quantity of the services provided. Every six months individual workers are rated by the district managers, who use their own criteria for assessment.

Comparisons of programs are rarely made at the national level, although specific innovations or new methods in providing care tend to be disseminated by the government. For the most part, information is shared on an informal basis when agency personnel meet occasionally at national meetings.

The evaluation of the home nursing care programs rests on the data collected by each local Cross agency. The forms completed by the nurses are analyzed at the provincial and the national levels and forwarded to the Division of Evaluation and Research at the national association's headquarters. The government similarly monitors these association records to make sure that the association adheres to program guidelines.

As stated earlier, the evaluation of individual nurses is done informally. In some areas, the head nurse talks monthly to each team member, while in other areas these informal discussions may be even less frequent.

The staff of associations within a given province may meet regularly to discuss plans and share new ideas. The national association meets regularly through various boards, along with other organizations such as homes for aged, hospitals, and the Central Council of Home Help, to further review plans for development.

MANITOBA, CANADA

The province of Manitoba operates a comprehensive system of home care covering both the social and medical needs of patients. All services are administered and controlled by a single agency, the Office of Continuing Care, but despite this high degree of centralization, regional differences do emerge as a consequence of local circumstances and inevitable adaptations. Some rural regions may assess clients and formulate treatment plans in stronger medical terms than urban areas, where both nurses and social workers act as case coordinators. Nurses are not trained in conducting social assessments and counseling. Consequently, regions that depend only on nurse coordinators design services with an obvious medical bent and fail to attend to the more complex social and familial problems of their patients.

Although the program is mandated to serve the growing aged population, the budgetary resources are not commensurate to the extent of need and may well be capped in the near future. Consequently, there is an inherent danger that both the program and its personnel will become stretched to the point where the quality of care is compromised in favor of quantity, and then the overall effectiveness of the program will be placed in jeopardy. The challenge to quality-of-care standards stems from the imperative to respond to the increasing demand on a nondeclining basis, at a time when resources remain constant. The strategical outcome consists of limiting services to their minimal or bare essentials. The costs of services must not exceed, except in special circumstances, those of equivalent services in an institution. Eligibility is similarly restricted to cases of stringent urgency, as determined by a coordinator and duly recorded on the standardized assessment forms.

As already stated, case coordinators are usually responsible for each client's care plans. However, for patients discharged from hospitals, it falls to the hospital case coordinator to draw the service plan for the first two weeks following discharge. The hospital coordinator monitors the implementation of the plan and visits each client regularly while maintaining contact with the specific care workers.

The home care program has instituted standards for specific types of care in its procedural manual, but there is no instrument for measuring the quality of care provided by the homemakers or home attendants. The performance of individual workers is appraised annually as a means of determining the quality of their work and awarding pay increments.

All continuing-care personnel are, in fact, evaluated on the basis of performance evaluations designed by the Civil Service for their respective positions and matched to their corresponding job descriptions.

The central office of the Continuing Care Program reviews each regional program annually, following formally defined standards.

Several criteria have been used in measuring overall effectiveness. Since the beginning of the program, the ratio of nursing home beds to the population has been reduced. Furthermore, the proportion of patients receiving light care in the nursing homes has declined from 20 percent to 14 percent, as these persons are now receiving care at home. Moreover, there has not been any increase in the number of hospital beds despite the fact that the proportion of elderly persons, and especially the very old, has increased.

The provincial government is reviewing the recommendations of a recent external review of the Continuing Care Program conducted by Price Waterhouse (1988). A primary concern identified in this report is the continual increase in the program cost.

The budget allocated in fiscal year 1986–87 to community care was CDN $24,000,000 while the amount spent was CDN $32,000,000. In 1987–88 the budget was CDN $33,000,000, but CDN $39,000,000 was spent, and for 1988–89 CDN $40,000,000 was allocated, and CDN $39,012,300 was actually be spent. Critics of the program see this as evidence that the program is "out of control." Supporters counter, however, that the amount actually spent was the original amount requested but the program is continually underfunded.

Related to cost considerations is the debate about a fee-for-service charge. Personal care homes (nursing homes) are permitted to charge a per diem of CDN $20.00 a day, but there is no fee for home care. The average cost of home care per year is CDN $1,500.00 per person, while care in a personal care home averages $1,500.00 per person per month. The per diem home care costs averaged CDN $6.60 in 1986–87, as compared to the lowest per diem cost in a nursing home of CDN $45.20 (Havens, 1987b).

In analyzing the cost savings of the home care program for the first month of a person's care, the financial savings are higher for those persons under sixty-five years of age than for older persons who require more services (Department of National Health and Welfare, 1982). However, home care is less expensive across the board than institutional services for the elderly, and it definitely saves the most in health and social service dollars per client.

Another recommendation of the recent external review report on continuing care was that a user fee for household maintenance services be applied. This would facilitate controlling the demand while also decreasing service costs. Again, opponents of charging for home care state that the costs of assessing and billing clients and trying to collect the fees outweigh the savings, because most of the elderly receiving the services would be able to contribute only a minimal fee in the eventuality that a sliding scale was instituted.

The program's policies and operations are being challenged, given the government's determination to control costs. There is a possibility that the service may revert to a stricter medical model and, consequently, assign a lower priority to social needs.

On the other hand, there are political leaders who believe the program should be expanded to new categories of clients, such as handicapped infants and adults who require a more extensive and continuous level of care. The system would then change in character from its present supportive features to a primary care operation.

Comprehensive evaluations of Manitoba's Continuing Care Program identify several strengths: the standardized assessment procedures, the single entry into the long-term care system, and its flexibility in meeting individual needs while providing for broad coordination between services. Additional strengths are the balanced recognition of social as well as medical needs and the absence of both time limits for the provision of home care and financial barriers to its utilization.

The main weaknesses are identified as the absence of a computerized data system, a poor financial base, excessively large caseloads, inadequate supervision, limited provision of respite and day care, and lack of specialized services such as speech therapy. Critics of the program underscore its deficient fiscal accountability procedures, while advocates and supporters claim its limitations stem from persistent funding shortages.

ARGENTINA

The physician dominance of the entire home care service in this country must be understood as a consequence of the oversupply of medical doctors. Argentina's free university education and generous admissions policies contributed to an overabundance of graduates in all the liberal professions. The market cannot easily absorb all of them, and in the case of physicians, many compromise by accepting disadvantageous contractual arrangements with the national health system or other medical insurance programs. Primary physicians are thus sorely underpaid, and since Argentina periodically undergoes cycles of rampant three-digit inflation, awaiting a three- to four-week reimbursement period could well represent a loss of 25 percent in the purchasing power of the outstanding bills. In sum, physician-centered home care prevails because physicians are a cheap commodity.

Primary physicians, for the most part, adapt to these economic realities by restricting their availability. Evaluators found that primary physicians conduct home visits only under exceptional circumstances, and even then they rarely follow up on cases. The quality of care leaves much to be desired. Older persons often have no alternative but to seek medical attention on a private basis even if they can ill afford it. After visiting a private practitioner, they rush to their primary physician to get the prescription rewritten so that it can be filled at no charge through their national health insurance coverage. Health policy analysts have observed that the fragile economic underpinnings of the national health program have reduced it for the most part to this prescription-writing component. Despite the promise of universal medical care, the age must still pay for full private primary medical care if they wish to receive quality, reliable services.

Homemakers and home nurses are also becoming scarcer, and it may take weeks until the prescribed and authorized first visit takes place. The national health program is in fact gradually reducing the scope of these ancillary services, in the expectation that families and neighbors will assume a greater share of care-giving tasks. Home hospitalization programs, for instance, hinge on the presence of a trainable family ready to be instructed by a home nurse.

Argentina's exemplary social policies have been thwarted by bad economic times. The country's crushing foreign debt, the costly Falklands war, and the recurrent trade deficits dictate inevitable cutbacks in social programs. Moreover, the three-digit rate of inflation further limits the real spending capacity of many of the country's services. The government has not modified any of the existing policies, nor has it reduced eligibility requirements or introduced copayments, premiums, or sliding fees as a means of stretching services. It chose instead to reduce the actual availability of services, home care included, by instituting a de facto cap on services. Limited services are offered on a first-come-first-served basis. There are no guarantees as to when people in need will actually receive them. The alternative to long waiting periods is to resort to the private or the voluntary sector. Argentina's model of home care services must be appreciated more for its intentions than for its accomplishments. In the absence of systematic program evaluation, policy analysts can only point to the gap between policy objectives and the program's actual scope and quality.

9

Summary and Recommendations

This study was prompted by the realization that the demand for community-based services for the frail aged and the disabled, such as home care, will be increasing relentlessly in years to come.

Despite these anticipated trends, home care remains a fragmented system with different funding streams and mutually independent agencies and service standards. Service gaps, cumbersome distinctions among workers' titles, lack of service continuity, stress, and poor working conditions result from this fragmentation. It is not surprising that turnover rates are high and that recruiting and training new personnel have become unremitting imperatives.

The goal of this study was to examine how other countries contend with such realities and whether they have succeeded in setting up viable and effective home care services. It sought to identify what could be learned from their programs and which aspects could potentially be adopted in the United States. A summary of the findings and the pragmatics of service delivery in the six countries is presented in the first section of this chapter.

THE MAJOR FINDINGS

The distinction between the functions of home health or home nursing, on one hand, and those of home help or homemakers on the other is well established, but the boundaries of these roles tend to overlap. Home-makers are increasingly assigned paraprofessional tasks drawn from nursing, occupational therapy, and social work. They include, among other things, administering and monitoring medications, initiating or planning leisure time activities, and counseling and advising about illness prevention and about activities of daily living. There is no explicit intent that homemakers turn into highly endowed generalists, but some planners do advocate a modicum of role diversification because it neutralizes boredom, enables the homemaker to attend to the client as a whole person, and fosters a greater sense of initiative in the worker. It may also reduce the need or quantity of routine home nursing visits. The trend towards greater syncretism and role blurring implies for the most part an upgrading of the homemaker, without necessarily causing a downgrading of the nurse and or home nurse.

A further specialization within the ranks of the homemakers is occurring, with generalists who attend to most basic activities of daily living and environmental needs on one hand, and heavy-duty specialists, who attend to tasks such as washing floors, windows, and bathrooms, moving furniture, and carrying heavy household or health equipment, on the other. The latter tasks are often contracted out to private providers. In one instance a national health insurance program subsidizes consumers so that they may hire heavy-duty task providers in purely private transactions, without the funding source's mediation.

Two models of organization of home care services are apparent. The centralized one is applied by governmental agencies, either at the national or the provincial level. Regional or county divisions and further smaller local and subdistrict offices respond to uniform definitions of tasks and formal regulations. This model has the advantage of uniformity of procedures and good coordination among services.

The opposite, decentralized model places most planning responsibilities on each local authority, usually a municipality or county, and its corresponding home care service. The central government establishes basic or minimum requirements but limits its input to collecting information and allocating subsidies. The local agencies have the autonomy of finding solutions to their immediate concerns. Decentralization has the advantage of increased flexibility and responsiveness to local needs. Workers are trusted and encouraged to act as problem solvers. Case review and service planning becomes a daily routine for teams of home care workers. Their supervisor is usually the case manager for the clients handled by the team. Team discussions facilitate and improve the case management function.

Coordination of homemaker and home nursing services may follow an assortment of service models. They may be both operating under the same public authority or agency. In such a case, a single supervisor, usually a nurse, follows up all cases and assigns homemakers and home nurses as needed, who, not uncommonly may work as a team.

In a second model, the two services operate independently. Coordination may take place in the form of occasional case conferences convened by either one of the services. There may be a routine or regular arrangement whereby the district home nurse meets weekly with the homemakers working in the same area. These meetings are not limited to case reviews, but may be also convened for consultation, prevention, and skills development.

A third coordinative model retains the separate administrative jurisdictions of the two services—the more socially oriented homemaker and the health-centered home nurses—but it gradually blends their roles at the field or district level. Services become a task-group responsibility shared by professionals and paraprofessionals. All workers must be ready to do whatever is needed at a given time. Team members must trust each other and undergo intensive training that includes inputs from all professional disciplines. They consequently spend many hours a week actually educating each other.

There is a plethora of case management models, even within a single country. Centralized administrative systems may designate care coordinators who conduct the assessment, assume the case-planning function, and enlist needed services—home care included—from their own agency or department. The coordinators have the authority to prescribe services without having to negotiate or recommend them to third parties. Once the home care service performs its duties, the coordinator monitors whether the services were delivered as intended, but lacks administrative authority over the service process. In a modification of this model, a community-based supervisor or coordinator is empowered with administrative authority over the long-term care staff and is authorized to shuffle resources among nursing homes, day care programs, sheltered housing, and home care. A third model parallels the latter but is hospital based. Case management is then combined with the discharge-planning function.

Case management may take place under the auspices of the agency that first has contact with a client. The case manager notifies the other services about any new developments or needs related to the specific client. Depending, however, on the developments of each case, one service may delegate case management responsibility to the other. In some programs, the case manager is selected according to the primary needs of the individual.

Coordination with hospitals may be initiated at the very moment of admission or close to discharge. In some instances the hospital head nurse contacts the district homemaker or home nurse supervisor to facilitate continuity of care. In other countries a special liaison nurse is employed to coordinate the discharge. In a third variation, an in-hospital multidisciplinary team that includes the patient's primary-care physician designs a new plan of care to be initiated at discharge. In the first instance, the hospital and home care service may rely on special teams of workers designated as "flying brigades" to attend to emergency situations when discharges have not been anticipated or properly planned. In the last model, which entails a multidisciplinary team, coordination is not really an issue, because the hospital itself operates its own continuing home care program.

Referrals to home care services may be initiated from a host of sources, such as discharge planners in hospitals, physicians, nurses, neighbors, congregate housing managers, relatives, and even the patients, or consumers, themselves. In most programs physicians are not required to be a part of the referral system. The assessment of need and the formulation of a service plan may require a full-fledged multidisciplinary team, the primary physician included, or just the area coordinator and a nurse or social worker supervisor, as often happens in more autonomous and decentralized systems.

The assessment itself may involve quite an elaborate instrument covering medical, clinical, functional, psychosocial, environmental, and economic issues, or it may consist of a rather expeditious set of open-ended questions. The simplest such questionnaire encountered in the study consisted of four questions: (1) What can you do for yourself? (2) What can't you do for yourself? (3) Is there anybody available to help you? and (4) What can we do for you? Some assessment instruments are standardized for an entire country, while others are designed by each local authority or agency, depending on the degree of discretionary power delegated to them. In some programs a simple assessment form is used for entry into the overall long-term care system.

Personnel may be recruited to home care services along a more fluid model that gives consideration to needs for part-time, supplementary income, particularly among middle-aged women, students, and even elderly retirees. Relatives and neighbors may be specially targeted if they live with or near the patient or client. The advantages are a greater sense of commitment and the possibility that these workers may be willing to extend their services to other persons in need. Local regulations may, however, require that care givers devote themselves full-time if they wish to qualify for a state allowance or compensation.

This model is crisis oriented, and consequently, more attuned to a wider range of potential workers. It accepts the reality of the workers' temporariness and will not, therefore, invest too much in extensive training. It admits to the relatively closed-ended, unskilled, and lower status of home care in an occupational market dominated by more upwardly mobile and more high-tech service professions. Finally, it recognizes that high turnover rates will continue, and consequently emphasizes aggressive outreach and recruitment approaches at the local or district level to ensure a steady flow of replacements.

In contrast, a more professionally oriented model seeks to upgrade the status of home care, in its diverse modalities, by instituting lengthier training, often starting in health professional high schools, and offering better pay, full-time employment, periodic retraining, counseling and support services, attractive health and pension benefits, and the semblance or promise of a career ladder. A concern, however, is that professionalized home care workers often emphasize the social and therapeutic side of their tasks to the detriment of more basic household tasks.

Regardless of the manpower model adopted, most national systems are heavily invested in retention strategies. Some of these include paid travel time, paid training time, clothing allowances, health leave days, psychological counseling and consultation, paid group support time, full fringe benefits for part-time employment, team rather than solo visits to clients' homes, team planning and rotation in household tasks, rotation between household and nursing home or senior-center duties, greater discretion and participation in services planning, in-service training (up to one hour of education for every three hours of work), and so forth.

Home care is viewed in most countries as a stage in the long-term care continuum that precedes or prevents institutional care. It then constitutes a discrete service in its own right, operating with its own administration and specialized personnel. Some national programs, however, are experimenting with the integration of all long-term care services in an open-care, or syncretic, model, whereby patients alternate between their homes and the nursing home, according to need, or move to the nursing home for short periods of intensive diagnostic and preventive care or rehabilitation treatment. They are followed by the same staff, especially by a home nurse that ensures the continuity of care between home and institution. There is no separate home care or nursing home personnel because the same staff rotates between home and institution in this open-care model. Home care and nursing home care are no longer considered distinct stages in a continuum, but one and the same service.

Home care's role in the continuum of services for the aged may respond to a total-care model that aims eventually to eliminate or limit the scope of institutional care. It rests on the principle that keeping the person at home takes precedence over all other cost-efficiency criteria. Home care would start out as the lead primary care service, but eventually become the dominant service. Requests for services would be offered, according to this model, on a nondeclining basis and according to individual need. This model tends to guarantee universal access regardless of income or type of disability.

A different model centers around the principle of complementarity. For each case, the program's primacy is conditional on the availability of other relevant services as well as on the presence of a viable informal support system. This model resists the trend to transform home care into total care.

A third model underscores health or medical interventions and consequently regards home care as part of either the primary physician's care plan or a hospital discharge plan.

The above-mentioned open-care, total-care, and complementarity models include, at least in principle, both health and social service components, but the integration of these elements is rarely a balanced one. Some national or community systems may give de facto preponderance to one over the other. Home care programs tend, in fact, to be more health- or medically oriented or controlled. There is, however, a growing realization that health-oriented programs usually treat an illness or functional condition but neglect the total person. Such programs also fail to properly include the patient in designing the care plan. Consequently, there is an emerging trend to add social services, such as counseling, leisure, recreation, and companionship, to these programs. Because many of the programs are administered by nurses, however, doubts are often expressed as to whether they are properly attuned and responsive to social needs.

Countries with comprehensive health insurance programs tend to extend home care services as a basic entitlement, usually free of premiums, deductibles, or copayments. The trend, however, is to require some participation in covering the cost of services, for instance, by means of a flat, nominal fee, a sliding scale, or a prepayment fee specifically earmarked for health and community services.

When services are offered through the public sector with literally no competition from private or independent providers, there is little incentive to institute quality-of-care standards. As the private sector begins to make inroads into this sector, the pressure to institute such norms— as well as licensing requirements—is mounting. Conservative political parties are advocating a mixed-service economy in which the patient or client has the freedom to choose from either public or private home care services. Where comprehensive health insurance programs are in effect, a system of vouchers would give the patient the resources to shop around in the service market.

This study was undertaken with the intent of reviewing selected countries' meaningful innovations of possible practical relevance to older persons, communities, policymakers, and service practitioners in the United States. By identifying different service models, it is possible to consider viable alternatives for transfer and adaptation. Specific recommendations for both a service model and guidelines for practice are made in the following two sections.

THE PROPOSED SERVICE MODEL: PROPOSITIONS AND AXIOMS

The proposed service model is based upon a series of propositions and axioms which provide a framework for policies governing home care. The propositions are as follows:

1. Access to home care may originate from diverse referral sources, including the client. It should not be restricted to a single gate-keeper or professional discipline.

2. Determination of eligibility, assessment, and preparation of service plans will take place at the community level, by a specially designated local agency. These agencies should abide by federal and state guidelines, but will be delegated the right to authorize the delivery and reimbursement of services.

3. Eligibility determination will take into account all needs of chronically dependent persons, including but not limited to their physical health and functional capacity. It will give equal consideration to social and environmental needs. The provision of services will not be contingent on a medical diagnosis or previous hospitalization, nor will it be reduced to short periods of convalescence or rehabilitation only.

4. A single standardized and multidisciplinary assessment procedure will be instituted for all long-term care services, not only or separately for home care.

5. Home care will be coordinated—through joint planning and the sharing of the same service teams—with acute-care hospitals, on one hand, and with day care, multiservice centers, congregate housing, and nursing home care, on the other. This coordination will facilitate a two-way transition whereby clients may go back and forth from their own homes to the nursing home.

6. There will be a single federal mechanism for fiscal coverage. Home care services will be funded with Medicare-related premiums. These funds could be supplemented with state and local resources as well with individual prepayments and/or copayments.

7. The distinction between homemaking and home health services

will be retained, but they will be placed under a single authority. Service plans will be designed by both services, and they will share many essential functions.

8. Clients will be assigned to a multidisciplinary team rather than to an individual home care worker. Teams of workers will have greater autonomy to organize and plan their work.

These eight propositions are in turn responsive to a series of axioms that define the policy framework, as follows:

1. Universal access to services
2. Decentralized administration
3. Standardized and multidisciplinary assessment methodology for all long-term care services
4. Primacy of chronicity as a determinant for services eligibility
5. Integration of health and social services
6. Integration of homemaker and home health services
7. Coordination of services with acute-care hospitals, long-stay institutions, and community services
8. Continuity and reversibility of service provisions between home care and nursing home care
9. Team approach in service delivery and greater decision-making latitude for home care worker teams

The propositions and axioms of the model are elaborated in more specific operational detail in the following guidelines for practice.

RECOMMENDATIONS FOR TRANSFER: PRACTICE GUIDELINES

Based upon the preceding analysis of services in the six countries as well as the postulated model, the following recommendations or guidelines for transfer to the United States are advanced:

—Home care should enhance the right of frail older persons to remain in their home environment. It should be more than just another cost-saving device aimed at preventing more expensive forms of institutional care. Home care should constitute, instead, the very core of a long-term care system.

—Home care should be considered a universal entitlement. Current restrictions should be reduced, and access to services should be facilitated by placing them under a single administrative authority. Funding should similarly be channeled through a single federal program, with supplements financed by the states. Clients' additional copayments should be graduated on a sliding scale basis, with a ceiling or maximum for any given year.

—The federal government should establish specific guidelines concerning costs, minimum standards, eligibility requirements, and copayments. Within this general framework, states and area agencies on aging should be delegated the authority to design services that are most appropriate for their target population. They should award service contracts to the private sector with the intent to promote competition while enhancing clients' freedom of choice.

—Eligibility requirements should be more attentive to the needs of a chronically ill population. Referrals for service, consequently, ought not be tied to an immediately preceding hospitalization.

—By adopting more decentralized features in the planning and administration of services, special attention should be given to visibility, outreach, and accessibility to services. Home care service offices should be located in closer proximity to their target population and should be able to respond more rapidly to requests for service. They should be designed in a way that assures equity of access and a broad range of services.

—Home care should transcend its dominant health care scope and also attend to the social needs of the frail person. This may be accomplished through specialized leisure and socialization services or by linking with adult day care or senior centers in the same community, provided that transportation and escorting services are also made available. Home care services should similarly be integrated in a single plan of care with a community network that includes nutrition, monitoring devices, prosthetic supports, and specialized housing arrangements.

—Home care services need to be considered part of a long-term care continuum. Service planning should be coordinated with acute-care hospitals, adult day-care services, and long-stay institutions. This coordination entails a single case-management process that involves hospital primary-care staff in the service planning task and uses a standardized assessment instrument. Continuity of care from hospital to community should be particularly emphasized.

—Assessment should be done by means of a universal instrument that taps all needs of frail persons. It should be used to determine all levels of service, not only home care, and it should be similarly used for periodic reassessments. Such an instrument may thus be used for discharge planning, case management, adult day care, home care, and institutional care. It should encompass the health and functional status as well as the psychosocial condition of the person.

—A long-term care continuum should be more than a sequence of autonomous services differentiated by their complexity or by the locus in which those services are provided. An open-care approach would make it possible for patients to alternate between services according to their changing needs. Thus home care patients could be placed in a nursing home for a short period of intensive treatment and then returned home. This preventive mechanism may postpone or even eliminate the need for lengthier institutionalization. If implemented, it will require an effective single entry and single case-management system with the authority to determine and obtain placement at any level of care. Similarly, it should have the authority to initiate financial compensation for all levels of care as well as aid for retaining the patient's home whenever this is judged feasible and cost-effective.

—Continuity of care between nursing homes and home care agencies should be established. By sharing personnel or forming a unified service, the same pool or team of home nurses and nurse's aides could assist patients. Workers, however, should be given the choice as to whether they wish to rotate among services.

—Payment to relatives may contribute to creating a more stable work force and reducing turnover rates. Such a program may be more effective than providing tax incentives, especially among low-income care givers.

—Career or occupational ladders should be created for home care personnel. These could be enhanced by training programs that define the upward progression from aide to supervisor to program director. Training should include ongoing staff development programs with mandatory paid attendance.

—Training should also be geared to multidisciplinary practice. It should prepare workers to share or exchange some common responsibilities, including functional and household assistance, and social and nursing care.

—Home care services should be provided on a team basis. Caseloads could be assigned to teams of several homemakers and nurse's aides rather than to individual workers. This would ensure that the workers know their clients well and allow personnel to rotate or substitute for each other when sick or on vacation, without causing disruption in the service.

—Teams should be delegated greater decision-making responsibilities. Together with their supervisors they should review each patient's condition, plan their own schedules, and make recommendations for additional services or needed supports.

—Home care workers should receive psychosocial consultation and backup services, particularly when having to deal with clients who are acting out or are otherwise difficult. Social workers, psychologists, or psychiatrists should be available to accompany workers in the field when needed to determine the best possible course of action with patients exhibiting serious behavioral problems.

—Training programs for home care personnel should be initiated and provided by regular academic institutions, especially by vocational or technical high schools and community colleges.

—Home care services should be offered not only to frail dependent persons living in their own homes but also to those living in groups or clusters. Reference is made here to small-group living arrangements similar to congregate housing, whereby five to six apartments with an equal or slightly larger number of residents are consolidated into a single service unit. This system has proven to work in some foreign localities because round-the-clock home care services can be concentrated in a more efficient way.

—Local home care agencies should offer emergency services similar to the "flying brigades" in other countries. The purpose of these services would be to fill circumstantial gaps or take care of unexpected situations or needs, particularly at the time of hospital discharge.

—Local home care agencies should create or contract specialized services for heavy-duty cleaning, home maintenance, escorting, companionship, and socialization.

—All elderly clients living alone who are recipients of home care services should be required to use a personal emergency response system, or lifeline. The lifeline should be connected to a central station that will alert the case manager's central office if the need arises.

—Home care agencies or area agencies on aging should conduct periodic community education and media information campaigns alerting the public to watch for prolonged absences and sudden frailty or bizarre behaviors among their aged neighbors. To this

effect, the agencies should institute a hot-line number for referrals.

—Home care agencies should coordinate with hospitals following
the discharge of patients to arrange the training of family members or informal supports who can assume some of the more complex technological tasks at home. The agencies should then
coordinate the tasks and schedules of informal supports and home
care workers in the performance of these tasks and establish both
formal and informal schedules of care.

References

Askham, J., Barker, J., Lindsay, J., Murphy, D., Rapley, C., Thompson, D., and Murphy, E. 1987. "The Home Care of Dementia Sufferers in Ipswich and Newham: The Guy's/Age Concern Home Support Project." In E. Murphy, ed., *Home or Away*, London: National Unit for Psychiatric Research and Development at the United Medical Schools of Guy's and St. Thomas Hospitals.

Audit Commission for Local Authorities in England and Wales. 1985. *Managing Social Services for the Elderly More Effectively*. London: Her Majesty's Stationery Office.

————. 1986. *Making a Reality of Community Care*. London: Her Majesty's Stationery Office.

Bass, S., and Rowland, R. 1983. *Client Satisfaction with Elderly Homemaker Services—An Evaluation*. Boston: Gerontology Program, College of Public and Community Service, The University of Massachusetts.

Berdes, C. 1987. *Warmer in Winter: Universal Long-Term Care in Manitoba*. Chicago: Center on Aging, Northwestern University.

Bergner, M., Hudson, L., Conrad D., and Patmont, C. 1988. "The Cost and Efficacy of Home Care for Patients with Chronic Lung Disease." *Medical Care* 26, (June 6), 566–79.

Bulau, J. 1986. *Administrative Policies and Procedures for Home Health Care*. Minneapolis: Aspen.

Capitman, J. 1986. "Community-Based Long-Term Care Models, Target Groups, and Impacts on Service Use." *The Gerontologist* 26 (August) 389–398.

Central Council of Home Helps. 1985. *Home Help Services in Practice*. Utrecht:

Central Council of Home Helps.

Chappel, N. 1985. "Social Support and the Receipt of Home Care Services." *The Gerontologist* 25 (February) 47–54.

Committee on Health Care Structure and Financing. 1987. *Willingness to Change*. The Hague: Information Service Ministry.

Department of Health and Social Security. 1976. *Priorities for Health and Personal Social Services in England, A Consultative Document*. London: Her Majesty's Stationery Office.

———. 1981a. *Care in Action*. London: Her Majesty's Stationery Office.

———. 1981b. *Care in the Community*. London: Her Majesty's Stationery Office.

Department of Health and Social Security. Social Services Inspectorate. 1987. *From Home Help to Home Care: An Analysis of Policy, Resources and Service Management*. London: Her Majesty's Stationery Office.

Department of National Health and Welfare. 1982. *Manitoba/Canada Home Care Study—An Overview of the Results*. Ottawa: Policy, Planning and Information Branch.

Dexter, M., and Harbert, W. 1983. *The Home Help Service*. London: Tavistock.

Doty, P., Liu, K., and Weiner, J. 1985. "An Overview of Long-Term Care." *Health Care Financing Review* 6 (Spring), 70.

Doyle, A. 1987. *The Myth of Homogeneity: Variations in Availability and Financing of Swedish Home Help and Institutionalization*. Jönkoping, Sweden: Institute for Gerontology.

Dutch National Cross Association. 1988. *Home Health Care in the Netherlands*. Bunnik: National Cross Association.

Eastaugh, S. R. 1987. *Financing Health Care*. Dover, Mass.: Auburn House.

Eliasson, Rosemari. 1988. "Perspectives and Outlooks in Social Science Research." Paper presented at the Dubrovnik Seminar on the Sociology of Science, May 9–20, 1988. Released by Stockholm's Socialforvaltning.

Ewanchyna, C., Collins, D., and Block, J. 1980. "A Ten-Point Model for Home Care Delivery." *Essence* 3 (Spring), 143–155.

Federal Register 44525, 44527. 1986. *Medicare Program: Criteria and Standards for Evaluating Intermediary and Carrier Performance during Fiscal Year 1987*. Washington, D.C.: U.S. Government Printing Office.

Glass, R., and Weiner, M. 1976. "Seeking a Social Disposition for the Medical Patient: CAAST, a Simple and Objective Clinical Index." *Medical Care* 14 (August), 637–641.

Government of Manitoba. 1974. *A Home Care Program for Manitoba*. Winnipeg: Division of Research, Planning, and Program Development, Manitoba Department of Health and Social Development.

Guntvedt, O. 1985. *Services, Housing, and Institutions for the Elderly in Norway*. Oslo, Norway: The Norwegian Institute of Gerontology.

Havens, B., 1987a. "Home Care and Day Care for the Elderly." Geneva: Prepared for Second Expert Committee Report on the Health of the Elderly, World Health Organization. (November 3).

———. 1987. "Manitoba Model: A Canadian Contribution to Emerging U.S. Long-Term Care Policy." Denver, Colo.: Prepared for Colorado Governors Conference on Aging, (October 16).

Heinz, John. 1986. "Letter to the Editor." *Pride Institute Journal of Home Health Care* 5, no. 3 Summer, 28–29.

Her Majesty's Stationery Office. 1988. *Community Care: Agenda for Action, a Report to the Secretary of State for Social Services by Sir Roy Griffiths.* London: Her Majesty's Stationery Office.

Hughes, S., Cordray, D., and Spiker, V. 1984. "Evaluation of a Long-Term Home Care Program." *Medical Care* 4 no. 22 (August) 640–651.

ICF, Inc.. Initial Formulation of the ICF Long-Term Care Forecasting Model. Washington, DC, ICF, Inc. November 1979. Cited in Meyer Katzper, "Modeling of Long-Term Care." *Human Services Monograph Series* 21 (July 1981), 66. Department of Health and Human Services, Project Share, Department of Health, Education, and Welfare Publication No. OS–76–130.

Kastelein, M., Dijkstra, A., and Schouten, C. 1989. *Care of the Elderly in the Netherlands, a Review of Policies and Services, 1950–1990.* Leiden: TNO Institute of Preventive Health Care.

Kastelein, M., and Schouten, C. 1986. *The Elderly in the Netherlands, Services, Systems and Policies* (draft version). Leiden: TNO Institute for Preventive Health Care.

Kent County Council Social Services. 1988. *Kent Guide.* Faversham, Kent: Kent County Council.

Klassen–Van der Berg, Jetha. 1985.*Achtergrondstudie vergrijzing, basisanalyse ten behoeve van scenario's over gezondheid en vergrijzing, 1984–2000,* Utrecht, Uitg. Jan van Arkel.

Kramer, A., Shaughnessy, P., and Pettigrew, M. 1985. "Cost-Effectiveness Implications Based on a Comparison of Nursing Home and Home Health Care Mix." *Health Services Research* 4 (October), 387–405.

Leader, S. 1986. *AARP, Home Health Benefits under Medicare: A Working Paper.* Washington, D.C.: American Association of Retired Persons.

Linzel, H. 1986. *Nota Ouberenbeleid in Flevoland.* Almere: Pvda-Flevoland.

Manitoba, Department of Health and Social Development. 1973. *Aging in Manitoba: Needs and Resources.* Vol. 9, *Special Data.* Part A—*The Elderly Population.* Part B—*Resources for the Elderly.* Winnipeg: Department of Health and Social Development.

Manitoba Health Services Commission. 1987. *Guidelines to Physician Services in Personal Care Homes.* Winnipeg: Department of Health and Social Development.

Ministerio de Acción Social. 1982. *Informe para la Asamblea Mundial sobre el Envejecimiento.* (Vienna, 26 July–6 August). Buenos Aires.

Nassif, Janet Z. 1986–87. "There Is Still No Place Like Home." *Generations* 11, no. 2 (Winter) 5–8.

National Association for Home Care. 1987. *Basic Statistics on Home Care.* Washington: National Association for Home Care.

———. 1988. *What Is Home Care?* Washington: National Association for Home Care.

National Council on Home Help Services. 1979. *Home Help Services in Great Britain.* London: National Council on Home Help Services.

National Cross Association. 1988. *Home Health Care in the Netherlands*. Bunnik, Holland; National Cross Association.

National Health and Welfare. 1975. *Report on the Federal-Provincial Working Group on Home Care Programs*. Ottawa: National Health and Welfare.

Office of Population Census and Surveys. 1982. *Nurses Working in the Community*. London: Her Majesty's Stationery Office.

Price Waterhouse. 1988. *Review of Manitoba Continuing Care Program*. 2 vols. Winnipeg: Queen's Printers.

Ratzka, A. 1986. *Independent Living and Attendant Care in Sweden: A Consumer Perspective*. Stockholm, Sweden: International Exchange of Experts and Information in Rehabilitation, World Rehabilitation Fund, Inc.

Rowbottom, R., Hey, A., and Billis, D. 1978. *Social Services Departments: Developing Patterns of Work and Organization*. London: Heineman.

Smith, Thomas B. 1973. "The Policy Implementation Process." *Policy Sciences* 4 (June), 197–209.

Sparer, G., Cahn, G. Robbins, G., and Sharp N. 1983. "The Paid Aid Demonstration: Summary of Operational Experiences." *American Association of Nephrology Nurses and Technicians Journal* 10 (Feburary) 19–29.

Special Committee on Aging. United States Senate. 1986. *The Crisis in Home Health Care: Greater Need, Less Care*. Washington, D.C.: U.S. Government Printing Office.

Spiegel A. 1987. *Home Health Care*. 2nd ed. Owings Mills, Md.: Rynd Communications.

Sundstrom, G. 1985. *Community Care of the Aged in Scandinavia*. Tampa, Fla.: The International Exchange Center on Gerontology.

———. 1987. *Old Age Care in Sweden*. Stockholm, Sweden: The Swedish Institute.

The Swedish Institute. 1988. *Old Age Care in Sweden*. Stockholm, Sweden: The Swedish Institute.

Szebehely, Marta. 1988. Personal communication on research in progress. Foubyran, Stockholms Socialforvaltning, Social Research Division of the City of Stockholm.

Taylor, M. 1986. "Letter to the Editor." *Pride Institute of Long-Term Health Care* 5, no. 2 (Spring), 24–25.

Trager, B. 1980. "Home Health Care and National Policy." *Home Health Care Services Quarterly* 2 (Spring), 1–103.

United States Government Accounting Office. 1986. *Medicare: Need to Strengthen Home Health Care Payment Controls and Address Unmet Needs*. Washington, D.C.: U.S. Government Printing Office.

University of Liverpool. 1986. *The Liverpool Intensive Domiciliary Care Scheme for Elderly Mentally Ill People*. Liverpool: Department of Psychiatry, Institute of Human Aging.

Zatterqvist, Marianne. 1987. *Personer Med Sjukvard I Hemmet Endygsinventering 1987–04–27–28*. Rapport fran halso och Sjukvardsavdelningen. Jökopings: Lans Landsting.

Zimmer, J., Groeth-Juncker, A., and McCusker, J. 1985. "Effects of a Physician-Led Home Care Team on Terminal Care." *American Journal on Public Health* 75 (February) 134–141.

Zwick, D. 1986. "Home Health Services for the Elderly: The English Way." In *Home Health Care Services Quarterly* 6, no. 4 (Winter) 13–65.

Index

About the Authors

ABRAHAM MONK, Ph.D., is professor at the Columbia University School of Social Work, New York, NY.

CAROLE COX, D.S.W., is associate professor at the National Catholic School of Social Services, The Catholic University of America, Washington, DC.